POWER OVER YOUR PAIN WITHOUT DRUGS

POWER
OVER YOUR PAIN
WITHOUT
DRUGS

NEAL H. OLSHAN, Ph.D.

RAWSON, WADE PUBLISHERS, INC. New York

Library of Congress Cataloging in Publication Data
Olshan, Neal.
    Power over your pain without drugs.
    Includes index.
    1. Pain—Psychological aspects.   I. Title.
BF515.044   1980   616'.0472'019   79-64205
ISBN 0-89256-108-4

Published simultaneously in Canada by McClelland and
    Stewart, Ltd.
Manufactured in the United States of America
Composition by American–Stratford Graphic Services,
    Brattleboro, Vermont
Printed and bound by Fairfield Graphics, Fairfield,
    Pennsylvania
Illustrations by Gail Schneider
Designed by Jacques Chazaud
Second Printing July 1980

This book is dedicated to
Mary, Sandy, Bobby, and Maureen
who are my inspiration,
joy and life.

◈

ACKNOWLEDGMENTS

I'd like to thank my wife, Mary, for all of her editorial comments, insights and patience during the writing of this book.

No acknowledgment would be complete without recognition of the contributions of Dennis H. Harris, M.D., who was instrumental in the development of the Pain Control Program.

Special thanks are extended to John P. Kelley, M.D., and Joseph R. Gottesman, M.D., for their technical advice.

I wish to thank especially the staff of the Center at Mesa Lutheran Hospital: John C. Merkel, Ph.D., Bill Arnott, M.A., Bernie Jarman, Ph.D., Barbara Greiff, M.C., Philip G. Sone, Ph.D., Don Miller; and Mary Lou Sargent, who keeps the Center running smoothly. Through the actions of these people the Pain Control Program improves each day.

Maryanne C. Colas, superior literary agent and friend . . .

Eleanor Rawson for her brilliant editing and constant faith in the book . . .

And my mother, Sarah Ruth Olshan, who, through her actions, taught me the true meaning of Pain Control.

CONTENTS

PART THREE

◆§◈

FOREWORD

PAIN! The warning signal of the body! At least, that's the way the medical profession has always been taught to view pain. It is only in recent years that medicine has begun to realize that there is a significant difference between acute and chronic pain.

Pain is the most common symptom bringing patients into a physician's office. *Acute* pain is a useful tool. It has a fairly rapid onset, lasts a relatively short time—hours, days, weeks—and subsides naturally or with treatment. It is a signal that something is wrong in our bodies and triggers many physiological and chemical changes that prepare us for emergency action.

Contrast this description with that of *chronic* pain. The typical "chronic pain patient" receives treatment but fails to improve. After weeks or months of various unsuccessful treatments, the patient is usually referred to another physician, then another, ad infinitum. While following this devious pathway, the patient often collects one or two scars from unsuccessful operations, becomes habituated or addicted to one or more medications, becomes physically deconditioned and increasingly involved emotionally.

Physical deconditioning occurs when the chronic pain patient permits the pain to become the center of his or her world. Social life, work, sports, personal relationships and other activities revolve around the pain. Activity and endurance decrease. Emotional involvement is a normal component of acute or chronic pain. The chronic pain patient is subjected to numerous failed treatments by several physicians, and is often told that the pain is "all in your head." He becomes increasingly frustrated, angry and anxious, then depressed. The patient often stops working and starts collecting some type of disability payments from insurance, Social Security, Workmen's Compensation or welfare. He becomes dependent on others, lowering his self-confidence and self-esteem and increasing his anxiety. Anxiety produces more pain, which produces more anxiety, which produces more pain—and on and on. We see this cycle perpetuate itself with a chronic pain patient.

Chronic pain has become an immense national health problem. It is the most frequent cause of disability in America today. Although accurate data is unavailable, we estimate that up to 80 million Americans suffer from chronic pain. The cost to the American public in medical expenses and loss of work productivity is greater than $50 billion annually.

A great deal of research has been undertaken in the field of chronic pain recently, and newer approaches are being incorporated in multidisciplinary chronic pain treatment centers. Though five years ago only a handful of such centers existed, today, they number over 250. New approaches to chronic pain have substantially increased the demand for these services, often leading to long waiting lists at these institutions.

Five years ago, Dr. Olshan and I founded Southwest Pain Treatment Center after we both saw the enormous need for such a facility. During the years that I have worked with Dr. Olshan, I have been impressed with the depth and breadth of his insight into all aspects of the chronic pain problem. Therefore, it is not surprising that he has assumed the much needed task of putting the chronic pain program into book form to make it accessible to the multitude who need it but who cannot travel to our Center.

This book contains many innovative self-help ideas and it is not only the first volume to provide detailed information regarding all aspects of chronic pain, but goes one giant step further by replicating the Center's complete Pain Control Program. This book will help you to gain "power over your pain without drugs."

Dennis H. Harris, M.D.

❧❧

PART I

❧❧

1

❧

Power Over Your Pain
Without Drugs

Paula K. was thirty-three years old, the mother of two young children. She worked in sales for a large department store and was proud of her promotion to department manager. There was only one drawback: her tension headaches were getting worse. As the demands of her new position increased, so did the frequency and intensity of her headaches. Paula couldn't afford to miss work, so she took large amounts of aspirin that only dulled the pain. A doctor confirmed the fact that her headaches were tension-related and suggested that she quit her job if the strain was too great.

The automobile accident wasn't his fault; the woman ran the red light. When he awakened, the doctors in the Emergency Room were standing over him. Herman's left arm was fractured in three places and it took the skilled technique of an orthopedic surgeon to repair the arm. Three weeks later, he was able to return to his job as an insurance salesman. The doctor gave him Percodan, then Tylenol #3 with codeine, then Darvon for the pain. After four weeks, the doctor said, "No more pain medication, just aspirin or Tylenol when the arm hurts." When the cast finally came off, the pain seemed to grow worse. The doctor said Herman would have to put up with the discomfort; most of it would disappear shortly, but a small amount could remain for a long time. He would have to learn to live with it.

* * *

Darrell always thought of himself as the type of person who would never become disabled. That was before arthritis struck. Within one year, Darrell changed from a man who was active in his retirement, playing golf and even jogging daily, to a pain cripple. Each specialist suggested his or her type of medication along with different therapies. Darrell tried them all, and although he did increase his level of activity, the pain remained: twenty-four hours a day, seven days a week, one year into the next. Percodan relieved a portion of the pain, but it left his mind foggy and Darrell spent most of his days sleeping. Late into the pain-wracked night, he would pray for relief.

Helen had stared in disbelief when the doctor told her that the mass in her left breast was malignant. The mammogram showed that the cancer had spread and the only treatment was removal of the breast. The surgery went well and Helen was home within three weeks. It took time to adjust, more than she had ever imagined, but Helen worked through the depression and the fears. She patiently waited for the pain to decrease and she grew frightened when it didn't. Her doctor assured her that no more cancer was present and that the pain was part of the healing process, something she should look on positively. Two years after the surgery, the pain persisted. Her doctors and others whom she consulted had long since stopped the pain medication. All of the doctors told her the pain was "unfortunate, but better than dying from cancer."

Laura was a twenty-eight-year-old audiologist who had suffered from headaches for six years. "My life was a mess, my marriage was failing and I was worried about losing my new job. I couldn't work with the headaches and when I took medications strong enough to help, I couldn't think straight. There were many times when I would sit alone in my office and think death might be a relief. I was so damned sick of going from doctor to doctor and no one could take away my pain!"

What's Left?

All of the people in these brief case histories were left without an effective method for reducing their pain. The stories are repeated in varying degrees, but all with the same basic message: *Chronic pain can destroy your life*. The Pain Control Program was developed as a response to the pleas of chronic pain sufferers, and for most who have used it at the Center, it has been a lifeboat in the sea of pain.

An Answer . . . the Pain Control Program

As the name implies, the Pain Control Program is designed to teach you to reduce and control the level of your discomfort. The program takes fourteen days to complete, but its principles will remain with you for the rest of your life.

As noted by Dr. Harris in the Foreword, less than ten years ago there were only a handful of pain clinics in the United States and now there are over 250 institutions dedicated specifically to teaching pain relief. Most of them charge thousands of dollars for a program ranging from two to nine weeks. But you don't need to spend thousands to benefit from the Pain Control Program in this book.

Later we'll go into more detail regarding the Pain Control Program, but for now let's take a few minutes and I'll tell you how the Pain Control Program was developed.

The Beginnings of the Pain Control Program

My interest in chronic pain began during my sophomore year in college with a twisting tackle that set my back on fire. After several weeks, the pain lessened, but it returned on and off. It wasn't until years later, at the coaxing of my wife, that I had an orthopedic surgeon check my back. I was told that I had an L4-5 nerve root compromise. I was given exercises to perform daily and was offered pain medication, but refused. There were times when I regretted that decision and yearned for "a pill" to take away the pain. I was told by my doctor that the pain would always be present and that I would have to learn to live with it.

I had just completed my studies for a doctoral degree in psychology, with specialization in medical psychology. At this point I met Dr. Dennis Harris and discovered that we both were interested in finding better solutions to chronic pain problems. My motivation was reinforced by my own suffering. We believed that answers could be found if we combined our two specialties of psychology and rehabilitation medicine.

Our Southwest Pain Treatment Center (the first in the United States) started as an outpatient program in Scottsdale, Arizona, but soon grew too large for the facility, so we moved to Mesa Lutheran Hospital. The hospital environment affords us an opportunity to provide inpatient as well as outpatient services.

Our program changed as we constantly revised our concepts of pain and suffering. I tested each technique on my own particular pain.

The Pain Control Program became multidisciplinary, involving self-hypnosis, autogenic therapy, individual and group psychotherapy, group exercises, physical therapy, occupational therapy, exercycle therapy and a lecture series explaining the principles of pain control. This program took place over fourteen days with a two-month follow-up. Although it was extremely successful, I felt something was missing. Most patients were getting from 10 to 35 percent pain relief. I used the program on my own pain and reduced it approximately 40 percent. But I didn't think this was enough. There was no reason why people couldn't be achieving 60 to 80 percent relief. An element needed to be added to our therapy.

That element fell into place when I learned about the discovery of a substance produced within the human brain that has painkilling qualities similar to those of morphine. This substance was given the name endorphin (endogenous morphine), the morphine within.

It was a miracle that was hard to believe. As I investigated it, I began to see the puzzle coming together. For the next ten months, we worked at developing a method that would employ the proven techniques of self-hypnosis and autogenics to activate at will these painkillers in the body. Ultimately, we developed an effective method of teaching Pain Control Training to victims of chronic pain, and it has proved remarkably successful in our clinical testing.

Why I Know the Pain Control Program Will Work for You

There are two reasons why I know the Pain Control Program (P.C.P.) works:

- I use it to control my back pain.
- Thousands of people have used the P.C.P. and found relief from their pain.

Patient Comments:

Ellen A., a former patient, said, "Before I started the program, I was just existing from day to day, but now I am able to live life!" Her comment is typical of the responses of people who have searched for as long as twenty-three years to find freedom from pain.

Another typical comment came from a twenty-one-year-old college student who was attending a local university on a tennis scholarship. He was injured in a motorcycle accident, lost his scholarship and had to work as a waiter to finance school. He was going to quit his job because of the pain, but his doctor sent him to me for treatment in the Pain Control Program. I saw him two months after he completed the program and the smile on his face reflected the results. "Before the program I couldn't work with the pain in my back, but now I have just a little dull ache and I can work all day. I have continued the Maintenance Program and I know eventually I'll be able to get rid of even the dull ache."

These are just a couple of comments of former patients who have used the P.C.P. Numerous case studies are included throughout the book, but now the most important case is You and how the P.C.P. can help You gain "power over your pain."

Some Common Questions People Ask on Starting the P.C.P.

How Long Is the Program?

The Pain Control Program is designed in a fourteen-day (two-week) format. By following each step, you will learn the techniques needed to control your pain.

You Mean I Can Do Something Myself?

Absolutely, this book *does not* contain the four Ms:

- Magic words.
- Miracle cures.
- Mysterious pills.
- Marvelous promises.

It *does* contain a proven method you can learn to help you solve your pain problems.

What Are the Advantages to Using the P.C.P.?

1. The treatment program can be used at home or in the office; it is completely transportable. Where you go, the program goes.

2. All of the techniques are noninvasive; in other words, you are not subjected to any surgical technique or required to take any medication.

3. The program is completely compatible with any medical treatment you are receiving.

4. The program allows you to maintain your normal lifestyle while improving each day.

What About My Doctor?

The book is not meant as a substitute for medical treatment. Remember, the people who enter our program have been referred by their physicians. Your doctor should be consulted to evaluate your condition and rule out any medically correctable problems. The P.C.P. is designed to be compatible with most medical procedures. You must not use this program as a substitute for medical counsel, but as an aid in your fight against pain.

Will I Be Pain-Free After Fourteen Days?

There is no guarantee how much you will be able to control your pain after fourteen days. Some people are totally pain-free, while others experience various degrees of relief. No matter how much relief you experience, I have designed the program so that you will receive continued and increasing benefit through the Maintenance Program. Reading the book is only the first step. As with any challenge, total commitment to the program will increase your chances of success.

Are There Other Benefits in Addition to Pain Reduction?

Yes. Most people who complete the program report: better self-image, weight loss, better muscle tone, increased endurance, improved level of activity, decreased anxiety-tension-depression-anger and, most importantly, a new lifestyle.

Why Does P.C.P. Work?

The revolutionary discovery of the brain's natural painkiller (endorphin) is the basis of the P.C.P. Each of us has the ability to activate the body's own painkiller and the Pain Control Program teaches you the method.

Can It Be Used for Any Pain?

Yes, no matter where your pain may be, the P.C.P. can be applied. This program has been used by people with:

· Arthritis	· Muscle Pain
· Back Pain	· Neck Pain
· Cancer	· Angina
· Neuralgias	· Facial Pain
· Colitis	· Sexual Pain
· Sciatica	· Postoperative Pain
· Ulcers	· Stomach Pain
· Causalgia	· Herpes Zoster (Shingles)
· Tic Douloureux	· Tension Headaches
· Raynaud's Disease	· Migraine Headaches
· Buerger's Disease	· Phantom Limb Pain
· Diabetic Neuritis	· Tennis Elbow
· Jogging Pains	· And Many Others

A Look at What's to Come

THE FOURTEEN-DAY PAIN CONTROL PROGRAM

Let's take a look at what's to come as we get down to the nuts and bolts of resolving the chronic pain problem. The fourteen days of the program are not meant to be a vacation; they mean hard work, perseverance and total commitment. I have planned each day for the utmost learning to help you in controlling and conquering your pain.

Each day of the program has been carefully designed in the following manner:

The Daily Lesson

At the start of the first nine days in the Pain Control Program, you will be given the daily lesson that includes information essential for your success.

Pain Control Imagery

This is the key to unlocking your pain. The daily lesson provides you with the skills to use pain imagery in step-by-step, learning-through-doing experiences.

Physical Reconditioning

Each day you will progress through the exercise program designed to increase flexibility, strength, and endurance; help facilitate weight loss; and generally improve your self-image. The physical reconditioning program is designed for the total you!

Keeping Track

Record keeping is essential. It affords you the chance to chart your successes and, I hope, inspires you to work even harder the next day. To help you, I have included the Pain Control Program Daily Record to be copied into your notebook and used each day.

The Three Assumptions

Before we begin, I have made three assumptions which are basic to your successful completion of the Pain Control Program.

First Assumption—that a qualified physician has evaluated your condition.

Second Assumption—that you will not use this program as a substitute for prescribed medical treatment, but as an aid in your fight against pain.

Third Assumption—that you will follow the program completely and thoroughly.

If you can confirm each assumption, you are ready to proceed to the Pain Control Program.

A Brief Word Before You Proceed

I don't expect the Pain Control Program to cure you of pain completely in two weeks. That's why I include the Maintenance Program to insure continued progress.

I have tried to make the steps as simple as possible while maintaining the highest quality, thereby giving you the best chance for success.

Throughout the book there will be self-administered tests, diaries and written exercises. I suggest that you purchase a notebook to record this vital information and your progress.

Remember, the true reward for following the Pain Control Program is gaining *power over your pain* without drugs.

P.C.P. + Commitment + Practice = SUCCESS =
FREEDOM FROM PAIN

2

❦

Pain... Man's Dilemma

BACKACHE	NEURALGIA	NECK PAIN
ARTHRITIS	BURSITIS	FACIAL PAIN
MIGRAINES	JOINT PAIN	CANCER PAIN
LEG PAIN		TENSION HEADACHES

These are just a few of the pains that afflict 60 to 70 percent of the American population. If you are like most people, you have already experienced one or more of these pain problems. If not, don't smile too quickly, for there is more than an 85 percent chance that within the next year one of these types of pain will strike.

The Cost of Pain

The impact of pain upon people is nothing new.

The actual cost of pain is devastating. Estimates run upward of $65 billion a year spent in medical care, Workmen's Compensation, lost wages and increased insurance costs. Unfortunately, most costs are passed on to us in the form of greater taxes and higher insurance premiums. One report estimated that roughly $10 billion are spent annually by pain sufferers for prescription medications and surgical procedures. Some experts believe that this figure may underestimate the true cost. It does not, for example, include the $900 million spent each year for over-the-counter painkillers such as aspirin and aspirin substitutes. The National Institute of Arthritis Research estimates that arthritis alone may account for 200 million workdays lost each year and $11 billion in medical care. In 1973 the state of California paid out $200 million in medical fees and compensation to people with low back injuries.

The Numbers Game

In addition to cost, let's look at the number of people whose lives are traumatized by pain:

- 25 million arthritics.

- 10 million people with low back pain.

- 40 million disabled people (ranging from mild to severe disabilities, but most in pain).

- 25 million people suffering from recurring headaches.

Why Do We Have the Chronic Pain Problem?

The chronic pain problem did not suddenly appear without warning. In my work I see certain factors contributing to the daily increase in numbers of people suffering from chronic pain. I have listed a few:

1. With advances in medicine, people live longer each year. Many diseases that terminated life at an early age are now kept under control through surgery and medication. By increasing our ability to survive to an older age, we have increased chronic degenerative diseases that are largely age-related and painful. The increased life span has, therefore, exposed more people to suffering for a longer period of time.

2. Heart disease and cancer are the leading causes of death in America, with accidents a close third. Many people injured accidentally would have died in the past, whereas with improved medical techniques, they now live out their normal

life spans. Unfortunately, a great number are *repaired* physically, but are sentenced to live with pain.

3. Stress-related disorders such as tension headaches, muscular discomfort, joint pain, hardening of the arteries, peptic ulcers, hypertension, sexual impotence, chronic fatigue and migraine headaches are steadily increasing. The inability of people to deal effectively with job stresses, family stresses and other tensions corresponds to an increase in chronic pain problems.

4. The increased use of prescription pain medications along with the preponderance of surgical procedures has caused many people to rely on outside sources for their own well-being. State compensation, insurance disability and other benefits to the injured worker have filled a need, but at the same time have rewarded people for being in pain.

What Has Happened to Pain Research?

When we compare pain research to other fields of scientific study, we find that motivation, financing and dedication have been seriously lacking. The International Organization for the Study of Pain is less than five years old and is still developing. Now that pain is gaining national attention, scientists who previously shunned pain control as a fruitless expenditure of energy are now showing renewed interest. But even that is not enough. There has to be an all-out attack on chronic pain. Why hasn't anyone ever had a "national telethon for chronic pain"?

What Does the Word Pain Mean to You?

How Does It Hurt?

- "It feels like my leg's on fire."
- "The throbbing drives me crazy."
- "It feels like the top of my head is going to blow off."
- "It's lightning shooting into my bones."
- "It's stabbing, like someone's jabbing me with an ice pick."
- "It feels white hot."
- "It feels like I'm tearing something inside."

Pain has been with us for as long as man has existed. The physical properties of pain have changed little since prehistoric man broke his finger while hunting for game in Africa's Olduvai Gorge. He grabbed his calloused hand, somewhat puzzled by the finger's crooked shape. He shrugged, grunting at the pain, and picked up his spear to continue to hunt. To him, pain was a way of life. The basic properties of a broken finger have not changed over the millenniums; what has changed is man's basic reaction to discomfort.

No two people react to pain in exactly the same manner. What may be a minor discomfort to John could possibly cause Frank to become hysterical. Early man did not have the convenience of doctors, clinics and hospitals, but research does show that many ancient civilizations used analgesic drugs on a widespread basis. Each society, culture or tribe has developed its own method for dealing with pain.

Searching for a Definition

Through my own experiences, I have developed a personal working definition of the word "pain." The words throbbing, burning and stabbing are familiar bedfellows. There have been nights when I have lain awake, not wanting to bother my wife, wishing that some magician would materialize and make my leg disappear. No magician ever appears and the leg is still there every morning.

My personal definition of pain does not apply to all of my patients with a similar injury. Since no two people react to pain in an identical manner, any definition must be tempered with the reality of each individual's experience and expression.

Finding a suitable definition is somewhat like trying to describe the smell of summer rain. Possibly this difficulty can be explained by the fact that in the brain the experience of pain is both cortical and subcortical. The cortical is the conscious part of our functioning and the subcortical, the unconscious part. The question of pain is further complicated, since part of the response takes place in a section of the brain known as the limbic system, which has been called "the emotional brain." If emotion did not play a part in pain, then developing a universal definition would be a hundred times easier.

The Memory of Pain

Each time you suffer from pain, the experience is recorded within the memory bank of your brain in much the same way that you preserve music on a tape recorder. At a later date, possibly under the same circumstances, the memory is recalled and you feel the pain before there is any insult to the body. In other words, the memory of old pain and anticipation of the new actually can bring about a pain response.

Archie Bunker's Example

Archie is walking along in his stocking feet and stubs his toe against a chair.

EDITH: "What's the matter, Archie?"

ARCHIE: (angrily): "I stubbed my toe! . . . AND HERE COMES THE PAIN!"

Just like Archie, someone who has previously suffered the searing pain of burning a finger on a hot stove may experience similar pain long after the initial injury is healed—whenever the hand is placed near a hot burner. The pain may return even if you only think about the hot burner. Your thought processes anticipate the pain and activate certain memory cells that can produce pain although there is no injury to the body.

The Two Components of Pain

The two components that comprise the pain experience are sensory pain and suffering. Each component has its own separate characteristics, though in some areas they may overlap.

(AS YOU READ THROUGH THIS CHAPTER, TRY TO APPLY THE INFORMATION TO YOUR OWN PARTICULAR SITUATION. Understanding the pain experience in terms of your own circumstances is a key to success in the Pain Control Program.)

Sensory Pain

This is part one of the pain experience: the response to injury or irritation, which relays information regarding the location and intensity of the noxious stimulation. Picture your nervous system as a complex electrical relay mechanism.

When you smash your finger, the sensory aspects of pain immediately send to your brain information regarding what part of your finger is injured and the intensity of the injury, and stimulate the reaction of pulling your finger away from the danger. All of this happens in *fractions* of a second; sensing pain is an immediate response, since often our survival depends on the speed of reaction.

Suffering

After the initial sensory aspect of pain (information) comes the suffering component, which is our reaction to the discomfort. It may come in the form of crying out, facial grimacing, fear, anxiety or other manifestations. Suffering has been described as the most complex and yet the weakest link in the entire pain response pattern.

The One-Two Punch

Many times the lapse between sensing and suffering may be only a matter of seconds.

(REMEMBER: SENSORY PAIN IS THE MESSENGER, WHEREAS SUFFERING IS THE REACTION.)

Some interesting studies, which are revealing about pain memory, have been conducted with patients who have had prefrontal lobotomies (surgical removal of the frontal lobe of the brain) for psychiatric reasons or for the relief of intractable pain, a procedure seldom used today. Studies show that after the frontal lobe of the brain has been removed, the sensation of pain may still be present but the suffering component may be significantly reduced. People who have had this surgery tend to live in the present and not become anxious about the past or the future, and have remarked that the pain was there but they didn't care.

Types of Pain

What Is Intractable Pain?

This type of pain is extremely resistant to treatment and in most cases has been present for over six months. For example, some intractable pain may arise from a back or a neck injury, from an amputated limb ("phantom limb" pain), or may be pain referred from other parts of the body or psychosomatic pains. It is a pain that does not go away naturally, but lingers, resistant to normal forms of medical treatment. The medical community has tended to use "intractable pain" as a catchall phrase to describe failures of treatment.

What Is Acute Pain?

Acute pain usually comes on suddenly and is directly connected with the healing process; in other words, as the injury heals or disease abates, the pain gradually lessens. Most acute pain does not last more than three months and is tolerable because it decreases over that period of time and is amenable to medical treatment. Acute pain may be extremely uncomfortable in the beginning, but over a short period of time the suffering and sensory components begin to diminish until they are no longer noticed.

A Case of Acute Pain

Ray D., a professional baseball player, is at bat and the count has gone to three balls and two strikes. He gets into his stance, bat held high over his left shoulder as he stares out at the pitcher, concentrating and waiting for the ball to be released. The pitcher goes through his windup and his arm flashes forward, releasing the ball at a speed well over eighty-five miles an hour. As the ball streaks toward the catcher's mitt, its rotation causes the small white sphere to curve to the left. In a split second Ray sees the ball and realizes that it is heading toward him. He quickly steps back, pulling his arms in close to him.

The move is too late, the ball strikes his forearm with a loud thud. Ray grimaces in pain and grabs his arm. There is a deep, stabbing sensation accompanied by a burning feeling down to his fingertips. He holds his breath, waiting for the pain to subside.

Several minutes later he jogs to first base, still holding his right forearm. A large bruise will follow; the pain in the forearm may persist for a while, gradually beginning to lessen, and by the end of two weeks, the pain will be completely gone.

What Ray suffered was acute pain. There was a sudden injury or insult to his body and pain developed. This pain would be considered chronic only if it persisted after normal medical care.

What Is Chronic Pain?

Chronic is the flip side of the pain coin. Many pain problems start out as acute and gradually assume chronic qualities. Chronic pain is described as any pain which lasts for over three months and does not lessen with conventional medical treatment, which might include surgery, drugs and physical therapy. I have seen chronic pain patients who have been suffering for as long as twenty-five years without relief. Chronic pain is why the Pain Control Program was developed.

How We Measure Pain

If I were to apply an exact pain stimulus, such as having you place your hand on a block of ice for a certain amount of time, your perception of when you felt pain and when the pain became strong enough for you to move your hand, would be different from almost everyone else's around you. Reactions that are similar are usually due to chance rather than identical pain response mechanisms. Scientists have spent years trying to define the elusive boundaries of each person's pain experience. At first they tried to categorize all people and if you did not report pain in a manner that was thought to be acceptable, then you were promptly referred to the local psychiatrist for analysis. The therapist assumed that there must be something mentally wrong with you if you did not report the pain experience expected by your physician.

A *Case of Chronic Pain*

When Marsha B. stopped at the entrance to the freeway a pickup truck suddenly slammed into the back of her car. Her head was whipped forward and then snapped back violently, leaving her dazed and in pain. Marsha went through the normal course of treatment, which included physical therapy, injections to stop the pain and exercises. One doctor suggested surgery to correct the problem. She didn't have surgery and went along with the doctors who told her that she had suffered a neck strain and it would take three to six months for her to recover.

One and a half years later, she was still experiencing pain; she was discouraged, frustrated and in constant discomfort. She had long since had to quit her job as a secretary and now received minimal compensation from the state. She hadn't gone out on a date in over a year; her social life was nonexistent. The doctor kept switching her pain medication, trying to find one that would work more effectively.

Finally, in frustration, he referred her to a psychiatrist who told her that the pain was psychological and that when she felt better about herself it would disappear. She left his office in tears and vowed never to seek psychiatric treatment again. Most of his avenues of therapy exhausted, the physician began to increase her medication, but this didn't help Marsha resolve the basic problem of her life's being slowly but surely eroded by the chronic pain. Marsha had joined the not too exclusive club of chronic pain sufferers.

We've come a long way since Marsha's time and most scientists in the field of pain will agree that each person's response is tempered by numerous factors, such as:

- How you were raised as a child.
- Genetic make-up.
- Previous pain experiences.
- Your environment.
- Psychological make-up.

Throughout the medical field there are scales to measure conditions in the body. A reflex may be 2+, eyesight 20/40 and on and on. The curious fact is that there is no standardized measure for pain. The patient is either in distress or not. We cannot hook up a person to a machine and get a reading of his or her pain index.

Since no instrument is available, the single most widely used method for determining your pain response is still the report that reveals how you *feel*. To help you determine this, I have developed a Pain Influence Scale and reproduce it below.

Please look it over and then test yourself. You should copy the questions into your notebook. No matter what your score, don't become discouraged; together we can change the results.

Pain Influence Scale

Rate your answer to each of the questions that follow on a scale of one to five, circling the value that best describes any pain you may feel:

1 = Not at all
2 = Very seldom
3 = Half the time
4 = Most of the time
5 = All of the time

Question One: Does your pain cause you to stay inside your house?

| 1 | 2 | 3 | 4 | 5 |

Question Two: Does your pain keep you from socializing with other people?

| 1 | 2 | 3 | 4 | 5 |

Question Three: Does your pain cause you to miss work?

| 1 | 2 | 3 | 4 | 5 |

Question Four: Does your pain cause you financial hardships?

| 1 | 2 | 3 | 4 | 5 |

Question Five: Does your pain interfere with sexual activities?

| 1 | 2 | 3 | 4 | 5 |

Question Six: Does your pain hamper or prevent leisure time activities, such as hobbies, sports, etc.?

| 1 | 2 | 3 | 4 | 5 |

Question Seven: Does your pain cause you to feel like an outcast?

| 1 | 2 | 3 | 4 | 5 |

Question Eight: Does your pain make you wonder whether your life is worth living?

| 1 | 2 | 3 | 4 | 5 |

Question Nine: Does your pain occupy most of your thoughts?

| 1 | 2 | 3 | 4 | 5 |

Question Ten: Does your pain cause you to become angry, frustrated or depressed?

| 1 | 2 | 3 | 4 | 5 |

Now, add up all the numbers you have circled and this will give you your pain influence score.

> 10–20 = Not much, but be careful
> 20–30 = The start of trouble
> 30–40 = Warning
> 40–50 = Danger, too much!

If your score is high, the techniques you will learn in the pages that follow will help you lower it. I advise you to take the test three weeks after you finish the program and compare the new score with the one taken before the program. Just seeing how much your score has dropped should bring a smile to your face.

But before we mount our attack, let's take some time to learn about pain threshold and tolerance.

Pain Threshold and Tolerance

Pain threshold is the lowest amount of stimulation needed to bring about an observable pain response. The observable pain response may be a facial twitch, a verbal shout, a gasp or verbalization of discomfort. Through my years of work with pain I've found that the pain threshold varies so much from one person to the next that it is an uncertain tool to use in generalizing beyond one individual. Researchers such as Dr. Richard A. Sternbach of Scripps Pain Clinic have used the concept to get a measure of the threshold of pain in individuals. Dr. Sternbach and his colleagues asked patients to squeeze a hand exerciser continuously while a tourniquet device was being applied to the arm. As a patient continued squeezing the hand exerciser, he or she was told to indicate when pain was first noticed. After the initial pain response, the patient was told to keep squeezing the device until he could no longer stand the pain (tolerance level). The patient's tolerance level is, therefore, that amount of pain which he or she can no longer stand. Through this experiment, Dr. Sternbach was able to measure an individual's threshold pain (when discomfort began) and determine that person's pain tolerance (how much pain the individual could tolerate). From this experiment you can easily see that there is a difference between pain threshold and pain tolerance.

A Sample Exercise

At this point in your reading I feel that it is appropriate for you to begin working with a sample of the Pain Control Program. To bring this home, I would like to tell you about how my wife used some of the Pain Control Program's techniques to overcome a problem she encountered recently.

Mary began to feel ill and developed a loss of energy, low-grade fever and chest pain. She immediately thought it might be the flu, but after it persisted for several weeks, she went to an internist and had an examination. The internist could find nothing wrong and thought that she might be working too hard at her job as a counselor at a community college. Mary slowed down, but the symptoms persisted. She went through long periods of frustration, depression and dismay over her increased and undiagnosed pain.

Finally, during a routine chest x-ray, a large mass was found in the lower right lobe of her lung. After several days, it was determined that the mass was caused by Valley Fever.*

The chest surgeon told her to go home and rest for two months. He also told her that if the mass did not become smaller, that part of her lung would have to be removed. Needless to say, the trauma of having a mass in her lung, combined with the constant fatigue of Valley Fever, left her extremely susceptible to depression and pain, particularly since her confinement occurred at the holiday season.

Mary was able to prevent pain from controlling her life, our marital relationship, our children and her relationships with her friends. Although she was in bed for most of those two months, she worked each day using the Pain Control Program.

Unfortunately, at the end of the two months the mass had not decreased in size and it was decided that part of her lung should be removed. The surgery was totally successful, but recovery from lung surgery is uncomfortable, and Mary continued to use Pain Control Program techniques during the very painful weeks that followed. Mary had been quick to stop taking narcotic medication, but she was able to cope successfully with the pain through the use of two techniques: (1) The Calming Reaction, (2) The Pain Drain.

I have included these two techniques as your first step to learning the basics of pain control. As with any technique, practice is extremely important, so don't expect immediate results.

Try the techniques. I think they'll work for you!

Technique One: The Calming Reaction

Carefully read the four steps to the Calming Reaction. Practice step three at least once every hour during the next two days. The Calming Reaction will soon become an automatic response to pain and will help to activate the body's built-in painkillers. Take your time and *don't* try to force the reaction.

Step One:

When you first feel pain, do not panic. If you panic, the pain

---

* Coccidioidomycosis—an infection acquired by inhalation of a fungus found in the semiarid regions of the southwestern United States.

will surely increase. Panic and tension only tend to increase the pain.

Step Two:

Don't let fear get the best of you. Calmly assess the situation. Be aware of where the pain is located, whether it is a new pain or old, and how severe it is. Try not to let your imagination get the best of you. Don't anticipate the worst! Statements such as, "I just know it's going to get worse, I can feel the pain getting worse already," should be strictly avoided.

Step Three:

Inhale deeply through your nose, try to take the air all the way down into your stomach and expand your stomach so that you fill your lungs completely. Exhale slowly through your mouth, trying to empty your lungs and stomach completely. As you exhale, your stomach should contract. Relax, and then repeat twice.

Now, inhale slowly through your nose to the count of two. Hold your breath to the count of three and exhale through your mouth to the count of two. Relax to the count of four. Repeat this pattern for several minutes. (You may find that using the count of three, four or five will be best for you.)

Step Four:

Get into the most comfortable position possible and close your eyes. Take a deep breath, holding it for a count of three and letting it out slowly for a count of three. Take another deep breath (count of three). Do this five times and on the fifth deep breath, as you inhale, repeat to yourself the words "I am." Hold the deep breath for a brief count of two or three, and as you exhale, say to yourself the words, "Pain-Free." The repetition of the words, "I am . . . Pain-Free" in sequence with your breathing, will immediately counteract the fear or panic that generally start at the onset of pain.

Technique Two: The Pain Drain

This exercise should be performed after you've used technique one for several days. Once you are able to feel a sense of relaxation through the breathing technique, then you are ready for the Pain Drain.

3

⋅⧸§⧸⋅

Chronic Pain Fallout

There is a great difference between the explosion of one stack of dynamite and the detonation of a nuclear bomb. The dynamite may cause severe destruction of property and life, but it is restricted to a specific area. The same does not apply to the detonation of a nuclear device. There is predictable widespread destruction, but the true terror of this type of explosion appears in the fallout. Radioactive debris can affect people hundreds of miles from the explosion. Acute pain can be compared to the stick of dynamite, while chronic pain, like a nuclear explosion, has its own fallout, which affects us physically and emotionally. If pain were an isolated sensation (explosion), then it would be fairly easy to deal with that experience without seriously affecting our emotional functioning. Unfortunately, chronic pain causes "pain fallout" that has far-reaching destructive effects on our lives.

The Shotgun Approach

In my years of treating chronic pain, I have found that most people who are experiencing pain tend to follow certain psychological patterns.

As you read through this chapter, keep a notebook at hand and record any comments that seem to apply to your situation. After you have finished the chapter, review what you have written in your notebook before proceeding to the next chapter.

The Spreading Epidemic

Would it shock you to know that the divorce rate among chronic pain patients is between 70 and 80 percent? The impact of pain is emotional, physical and economic.

No one can predict exactly what changes will accompany the pain, but identifying your own emotional component is the first step to stopping chronic pain fallout.

Looking at Yourself

Mary Lou came into my office a shaken woman. Her doctor had recommended the Pain Control Program. I spent time explaining the program, but when I got to anything touching on the psychological she would become angry and say, "I hope you don't think this is just imagination. I'm not some kind of nut!"

I reassured Mary Lou that we in no way thought she was mentally ill, but I did explain to her about pain fallout. She was immediately more receptive to my suggestion that she take The Fallout Profile. I'd like you to reproduce the same profile in your notebook before we go any further.

The Fallout Profile

Do any of the characteristics listed below apply to you at this time?

- Decreased tolerance for pain.
- Increased fatigue.
- Insomnia (difficulty sleeping).
- Inability to concentrate or poor concentration.
- Increased feelings of guilt.
- Reduced sexual interest or activity.
- Increased anxiety.
- Increased irritability.
- Thoughts of suicide.

Make a note of those that do. To get a better understanding of your pain fallout, move on to the explanations and case histories provided for each statement that describes your condition. Can you see yourself in any of these examples?

1. Decreased Tolerance for Pain

You begin to notice that your ability to tolerate certain amounts of pain has decreased. Before you had the chronic pain, a mild headache would have been a small distraction of little concern. But now your tolerance for pain has decreased and that minor headache becomes unbearable. Your tolerance for the chronic pain problem grows less and less as you struggle for some relief.

CASE

Harry K. closed his eyes and clenched his teeth, trying to keep from yelling. His toe felt as if it were going to explode. Finally, he screamed out at his young son who had inadvertently ridden the bicycle over his foot. Harry's toe still hurt him and now he felt the guilt of yelling at his son for something that had been an accident. Before Harry's back injury, an incident such as this would have brought about the same amount of pain, but his reaction would have been much different. Anger and frustration would not have played such a role in the pain reaction. With his pain tolerance lowered, the anger increased the feelings of discomfort.

2. Fatigue

You either tire easily or feel fatigued most of the time. You lack the motivation for trying new things or finishing old projects. Your amount of sleep does not make any difference, for eight hours may not overcome the mental and physical fatigue that chronic pain brings about. Because of the fatigue, you tend to give up easily and feel depressed.

CASE

Doris S. suffered from arthritis. Although in constant pain, she got eight hours or more of sleep during the night, but by ten o'clock the next morning she was ready to return to bed. "I can't understand it. I get a good night's sleep but by the middle of the morning I'm so tired I just want to get back in bed. Many times I go back to sleep and get up around two in the afternoon, but by five o'clock I'm exhausted and go back to sleep. My family must think I'm a big fake. My husband is really kind, but I know he gets angry when we can't go anywhere because I'm either in pain or too tired!"

3. Insomnia

Although sleep may be desired and needed, it becomes elusive. Even if you are able to fall asleep, you may awaken several times during the night, thus leaving yourself with a feeling of sleep frustration by the morning.

CASE

Mary M. suffered from chronic tension headaches. When she reported problems with sleep to her physician, he prescribed a medication to be taken before bedtime. This medication worked, but worked so well that she felt drowsy and hung over in the morning. Her physician tried several other drugs, but all of them gave her the same reaction. Without medication, she would toss and turn, trying to fight her way into sleep, usually without success. The more she struggled for sleep, the worse her headaches would become. Finally, in complete exhaustion, she would drift off into an uneasy sleep, usually awaking several times during the night to repeat the process. Lack of sleep added to her tension headache problems and soon Mary was sleeping for only two or three hours each night. Before Mary knew it, she was taking more and more drugs and wondered if a good night's sleep would ever be possible without a headache or medication.

4. Inability to Concentrate

Constant pain definitely hampers your ability to retain information. After watching a television program or reading a book, you find it difficult to remember what went on. Your mind always seems to drift back to the pain.

CASE

Kathy W. had followed her favorite soap operas closely for over two years, but since her neck injury a year and a half ago, she was finding it increasingly difficult to remember what happened in the previous program. While she was watching television, her mind would wander, always focusing on her pain. The same thing would happen when she read an article in a magazine; she could understand the content, but five minutes after reading the story she was hard pressed to remember what it was about. She was beginning to think that she must be going crazy!

5. Guilt

This emotion is frequently present when you have chronic pain. There is significant build-up of guilt regarding: inability to maintain employment, financial impact upon your family, inability to participate in family activities and impaired sexual activity. Guilt associated with chronic pain is like a snowball rolling downhill. It starts out very small, but as it gains weight and momentum, it wreaks havoc on anything in its path.

CASE

"To me, guilt is like a cancer. Once it attacks you, it spreads and spreads until it finally kills you." Ray D. was serious when he described his feelings about the guilt he felt due to his arthritis. "I don't even feel like a real man. It is such a horrible, helpless feeling." Ray was referring to his inability to work. Sex with his wife was rare because of the pain, and guilt had become a double-edged sword cutting away at his life.

6. Reduced Sexual Interest and Activity

The person who is in chronic pain may experience a reduction in sexual interest. When you're in pain, sexual activity and sexual desire seem to take a real nose dive. The pain occupies so much of your thought process that anything concerning sex has difficulty breaking through the pain barrier. And if you do manage to break through the barrier, then the pain you experience during sexual activities may cause you to think twice before you have sex again. From lack of interest and fear of pain, such problems as impotency in men and inability to achieve orgasm in women may develop.

CASE
Richard D. first began to notice his avoidance of sex eight months after the automobile accident. The injury to his back had not healed properly and whenever he and his wife engaged in intercourse, he would experience pain almost immediately and the next morning his back would be so stiff and tight that he couldn't straighten up. He was caught in a double bind: if he took pain medication, then his ability to perform sexually decreased, but if he didn't take the medication, the pain killed any chances for enjoyment or orgasm. He was too embarrassed to tell his wife and decided the best thing to do was to try to avoid sex totally. His wife was confused by his behavior and tried to talk to him, but he refused to discuss the situation. His wife was at a loss to understand his behavior and assumed he must have lost interest in her as a woman.

7. Increased Anxiety
Chronic pain is usually accompanied by an increase in anxiety and tension. If your pain is not resolved, you will be caught in a vicious circle of chronic anxiety that causes actual physical changes (see Chapter Five). The longer your chronic pain persists, the more chronic anxiety becomes a part of your total emotional make-up.

PAIN . . . TO . . . ANXIETY . . . TO . . . INCREASED TENSION . . . TO . . . INCREASED PAIN.

CASE
Susan K. knew she was an emotional mess. The harder she tried to relax, the more unsuccessful she was, experiencing only an increase in her anxiety and pain. She was anxious about the continued pain, the financial problems, the family situation, reinjury and what would happen in the future. When she wasn't thinking about the pain, she

was worrying about whether she would ever be able to return to work. With two young children and an ex-husband who did not send child support regularly, the future seemed bleak.

8. *Irritability*

People who suffer from chronic pain usually show increased signs of irritability as they struggle to find relief. After going from one doctor to the next, one medication to the next and even one surgery to the next, you may find yourself becoming more irritable and frustrated each day.

CASE

"Even the slightest sounds send me into orbit. I know I'm jumping all over my children when I really shouldn't." Ruth wiped the tears from her eyes as she described the increasing irritability she felt when no one was able to help her get rid of her headaches. She knew what was happening, but didn't know how to stop it.

9. *Thoughts of Suicide*

I have found that people who are caught up in the web of chronic pain frequently have thoughts of suicide. There is no accurate data relating to how many people with chronic pain actually take their lives through an overdose of medication, automobile suicide or other unverifiable means. Sometimes hopelessness reaches such a level that people feel the only escape from chronic pain is death.

CASE

Rachel S. felt that suicide was the only way left to get rid of her pain. Two back operations, numerous medications and, finally, addiction to codeine left her feeling that life contained no more meaning. When I saw her in the hospital after an attempted overdose, I was struck by her question to me. "Nothing has worked for my pain; my husband has left me; I no longer have a job; when I look in the mirror I don't know whose reflection is staring back at me, I look so old. Give me one good reason why I should go on living! Life isn't worth living with this pain!"

THERAPY THOUGHT: *All of the people mentioned in these case studies have since gone through the Pain Control Program and have returned to a better way of life. But you cannot control chronic pain fallout unless you are willing to take the risk of learning more about your behavior.*

Pain Payoffs

The first step is to learn about the effect of pain fallout. The second is to discover any hidden pain payoffs you may unconsciously lean on. It is difficult to admit to yourself that you are getting some payoff for your pain. When I look back at my own pain, I realize I was getting some payoffs, but it would have been difficult to admit this to myself. When I finally did realize what was happening and changed my behavior, pain control was easier.

Pain payoffs originate in our younger years. This is a time when we learn to manipulate through sickness. When we're sick we don't have to go to school, people seem nicer, less is required of us and more attention is dispensed by all concerned. As we grow up, each of us retains a small portion of that child who gets a payoff for being sick. When we experience pain, the child tends to reappear. For most of us, the payoffs are at an unconscious level and we may not be aware of them.

Three Payoffs

Three types of payoffs are usually seen when someone suffers from pain over an extended length of time. These are by no means all of them and I'm sure you can think of others, especially if you are in pain yourself. I call these three payoffs CAM: Center Stage, Avoidance and Monetary Advantage.

1. Center Stage

Just like an actor standing on center stage, the individual who reports pain receives the immediate attention of those around him. The pain sufferer eventually has his center stage syndrome reinforced by the simple fact that the more he complains, the more attention he receives. This technique is used on relatives, children, spouses and even the patient's physician. The complaint of pain becomes a manipulation to gain increased amounts of attention that the patient feels justified in receiving. Many people with whom I have dealt have the center stage syndrome without being fully aware of its presence. The danger of this syndrome occurs when pain behavior is exhibited long after a decrease in physical symptoms. A pattern of pain behavior becomes programmed into the brain in an attempt to gain more attention.

CASE

Harold S. sprained his lower back while lifting a sack of fertilizer in the backyard. The doctor recommended bed rest and muscle relaxants. After two weeks in bed, Harold's pain had decreased significantly but a new behavior had developed through his "center stage syndrome." After the initial injury, his wife and two daughters waited on him continuously, providing anything he needed. At first the attention was overwhelming, but he soon began to like it and quickly learned that the more pain he reported, the more attention he received. By the end of the second week his back had improved, but his reports of pain continued to increase. He was becoming a star of the center stage syndrome.

2. Avoidance

It is an ingrained part of human nature to avoid stressful situations. If you are in pain, this avoidance behavior is easier to achieve. Pain becomes the excuse for avoiding responsibility and may also be used as a justification for defeat and failure.

RESPONSIBILITY . . . TO . . . AVOIDANCE . . . TO . . . INCREASED STRESS . . . TO . . . INCREASED PAIN.

CASE

Sylvia C. felt an increase in headaches whenever she had to take a test. The pain became her mechanism for avoidance, and even after graduation from college she maintained this behavior in her work situations. When she was faced with making a speech to a sales group, she used an excuse of pain to be absent and therefore avoid the stressful situation and also the possibility of performing poorly. The avoidance behavior began to have a contagious effect and soon she was using pain to avoid even minor stressful situations, such as balancing her checkbook, completing reports at work, social interactions or dating, just to name a few.

3. Monetary Advantage

The monetary return from pain is a topic avoided by most people with pain or treating pain. I have had occasion to see patients who had numerous disability policies and were actually making more money while away from work than they would have been making if they had returned to their former employment. Unfortunately, our society is caught in a double bind by the way that pain problems are reinforced by supplementary income from local and federal agencies. It has been my experience that most of these programs are poorly administered, and abuse, intentional and unintentional, is quite widespread. Often the compensation is a very poor and ineffective substitute for rehabilitation.

CASE

Merle was twenty-three years old when first injured. A meat cutter by trade, the back injury prevented him from returning to work for over a year. When I first saw him at the clinic, he seemed sincere in his desire to learn how to control his pain. As the Pain Control Program progressed, it became obvious that Merle was just going through the motions. I confronted him with this and he angrily denied any malingering behavior. The next day I confronted him again and received the same denial. That afternoon, after a long discussion, he finally admitted that he was in the program only because the insurance company had insisted. With some bravado, he informed me that by combining the monthly compensation check with disability payments, his monthly income (tax-free) was four hundred dollars more than when he was working. "Why should I get better? There's no profit in it," he said. That afternoon was his last day in the Pain Control Program.

Discovering Your Payoff

Discussing pain payoffs is not easy, for I honestly believe that most people are not consciously striving for any payoff. If you are totally honest with yourself, you will probably find that you are receiving some type of payoff, whether major or minor. Large or small, pain payoffs work in direct opposition to your learning to control pain.

If these payoffs operate at an unconscious level, then, you may ask yourself, "How will I know if I have pain payoffs?" The answer is quite simple. I have developed the Payoff Index, and after you answer these questions, your score will tell you whether there is a payoff component to your pain. I'd like you to reproduce the Payoff Index in your pain notebook before taking the test.

The Payoff Index

On a piece of paper please answer the following questions by placing the appropriate number describing your pain in a column.

1 = Never
2 = Seldom
3 = Sometimes
4 = Always

1. Does your pain increase under stress? _____
2. Do you get special privileges for being in pain? _____
3. Do you get more attention since you have been in pain? _____
4. Is your pain the main topic of discussion among family and friends? _____
5. Do you use pain as an excuse to get out of work? _____

Now total your scores for all of the questions. Here is the prognosis for your chances of having a pain payoff:

> 5–10 = MILD pain payoff. Probably only affects your pain slightly.
>
> 10–15 = MODERATE pain payoff. Beware of those payoff behaviors that may be hindering your ability to reduce pain.
>
> 15–20 = DANGER. Your chances of becoming "pain free" are being severely restricted unless you make an effort to change the payoff behaviors.

Note: I AM IN NO WAY SAYING THAT A HIGH PAYOFF SCORE INDICATES THAT THE PAIN IS PSYCHOLOGICAL. I AM SIMPLY SAYING THAT A HIGH SCORE INDICATES THAT A PAIN PAYOFF MAY BE ONE OF THE FACTORS MAINTAINING YOUR PAIN AND ADDING TO YOUR SUFFERING.

The Six Laws

If your Pain Payoff Index is not good, don't moan and groan, but try using the six laws of pain behavior. Take the time to write them in your notebook, and while you're at it, write them on a piece of paper to keep in your wallet or purse. Read them at least several times a day; believe them and use them:

· Don't talk about your pain!
· Don't use pain as an excuse!
· Don't use pain to get out of your responsibilities!
· Don't let anyone become a professional nurse to you!
· Don't use pain to manipulate others!
· Don't be helpless/hopeless . . . always be positive!

Helpless/Hopeless

Let's not forget those helpless/hopeless feelings that attack anyone who suffers from chronic pain. "You've got to keep hope," is a statement most people in pain hear over and over again, but no one bothers to tell them how to maintain hope. These feelings of hopelessness/helplessness may be increased by the pressures of society's expectations. Society places numerous demands on us and dictates how we should react to pain. Some of these are:

- · Women are expected to endure the pain of childbirth.
- · Men are expected to be tough and not cry when they are hurt.
- · Adults are expected to endure pain better than children.
- · All pain should be avoided.
- · If no physical reason for pain can be found, then you must be crazy.
- · Athletes can stand more pain than other people.
- · People in pain should be pampered.
- · Doctors are the only people who can take the pain away.

I'm sure that you can think of more statements but these should provide you with examples of how societal pressures partially determine our reaction to pain. These unwritten laws may serve as your ticket to a ride on the merry-go-round of suffering and, once on, getting off can be an extremely difficult task.

The Vicious Cycle of Pain

The vicious cycle of pain is simple and, like a weed, takes very little nourishment to grow into a sizable menace. It is important for you to know about it, now, for the Pain Control Program is designed to teach you how to break that cycle.

A Typical Pain Cycle

Pain . . . Frustration . . . Depression . . . More Pain . . . Medication . . . More Pain . . . Anger . . . Increased Medication . . . Habituation or Addiction . . . Increased Irritability . . . Increased Depression . . . More Doctors . . . Possible Surgery . . . Lower Tolerance to Pain . . . Increased Medication . . . Increased Depression . . . Increased Frustration . . . and the Cycle Closes, Leaving You with More Pain and No Way off the Merry-Go-Round.

Starting to Fight the Fallout

We've spent a lot of time talking about chronic pain fallout and the vicious cycle. Now let's take a look at chronic pain's flip side: depression.

Up from Depression!

"I feel so depressed, I'm going to stay in bed until the pain goes away." That statement was made by a twenty-four-year-old woman who came into my office at the insistence of her husband. She had a classic case of chronic pain depression. Two back operations and a complete merry-go-round of narcotic medications proved completely unsuccessful. Most of her days were spent in bed, languishing in her own depression, convinced that she would feel better only if her pain were totally gone.

Like many people who suffer from pain depression, she was essentially inactive, waiting for someone to come along, wave a magic wand and take away all of her pain for her. The thought of actively participating in her rehabilitation never crossed her mind. The lack of any meaningful physical, social or recreational activities only caused her to sink deeper into depression.

Hand in Hand

As pain increases, in intensity, frequency or duration, depression does the same. The opposite is also true; if you decrease your depression, perception of pain will also decrease.

Here are some typical depressive statements. See how many are similar to what you say to others or to yourself.

> "I just can't seem to sleep anymore."
> "I don't feel good about myself."
> "I can't seem to think straight anymore."
> "I feel listless."
> "Nothing seems to interest me anymore."
> "I don't like being around other people."

"I feel like I'm in a deep rut."
"I can't get along with anyone anymore."
"I feel like I'm in a daze."
"Nothing will ever work out."

How many of the statements apply to you? If the "depression shoe" fits, DON'T wear it! Try the five steps for overcoming pain depression.

Step One: Increase your level of activity. Get away from the television set and do something physically active, whether it's walking around the block, going window shopping or going for a bicycle ride. Force yourself off your seat and into activity. Pick an activity you are physically capable of, something you like, and repeat it often.

Step Two: Stay away from other people who are depressed. This means phone calls or direct conversations. If you have a friend who constantly calls you with depressing news inform her or him that you no longer receive such phone calls. Try to surround yourself with people who are not depressed.

Step Three: Realize that the more you worry about depression, the worse it will get. Depression is like quicksand; the more you struggle, the deeper you sink. Don't fall into the trap of focusing your entire life on depression.

Step Four: Make a list in your notebook of "up" things you can do, and if you should feel depression beginning, take out the list and go through the items. Substitute activities that make you happy for depressive thoughts.

Step Five: Remember that depression is only a state of mind, but a state that affects the body. One of the best remedies for depression is laughter. If you can laugh, then you have one of the most powerful psychological antidotes for the "slump" and you can use it, free of cost, without a prescription and without danger of overdosing. Depressed people should not go to depressing movies, watch depressing programs on television, read depressing books, and many times they should refrain from listening to, watching or reading depressing news. Try watching a movie that you know will have a happy ending or reading a book that has an uplifting theme.

Actively concentrating on removing depression from your life is an excellent first step toward preparing yourself for the Pain Control Program.

4

⋰⧈⋱

The Drug Merry-Go-Round

He was addicted to Percodan and after five years of taking massive doses of the narcotic, he contemplated suicide. He related a frightening tale of manipulating doctors into prescribing higher dosages of narcotic painkillers. The pain from his neck injury had caused devastating emotional changes. But a deeply buried desire to live stopped him, and at that point he made the decision to seek help. The man I've just described is Jerry Lewis, and his battle with chronic pain and painkiller addiction could be the rule rather than the exception.

You may wonder why I've started this chapter with an example of a well-known performer, and my answer is quite simple: no one is immune from chronic pain, and more importantly, chronic pain can lead to drug addiction, a legalized road to disaster. Jerry Lewis's story is repeated literally thousands of times daily in the United States alone. His public disclosures may have helped countless sufferers face the reality of their pain medication problem.

As you read this chapter, at no time should you alter your own medication without seeking advice from a physician. Most of my patients have found that after completion of the Pain Control Program, they are capable of substituting nonnarcotic medications for narcotics and in many instances refrain from taking pain medication at all. Always remember that your doctor may be prescribing pain medication in direct proportion to how much you complain about the pain. Most doctors are quite pleased if you say that you are controlling your pain more effectively and would like to reduce the amount of drugs you are taking. Doctors are very aware of the problems created by narcotics such as Percodan, which Jerry Lewis took, but often they are at a loss to provide methods for reducing the pain when drugs or surgery have not been effective. Physicians have been trained to consider analgesics as a treatment of choice for pain.

Analgesics

Analgesics are any medication that raise your threshold of pain. They in no way cure the pain problem, they simply increase the amount of pain you can comfortably withstand. Analgesics, therefore, have one major role and that is to reduce your perception of pain. Their period of effectiveness depends upon the type and intensity of pain but may last from one to ten hours.

The Problem with Analgesics

Analgesics have several basic problems. The body will gradually become accommodated to a specific drug and after a period of time larger doses will be needed to gain the same effectiveness. Extended use of narcotic analgesics can lead to addiction. Even the most powerful analgesic only masks the pain and when the drug is no longer in your bloodstream, the pain returns. For numerous people in pain, the only answer is to take analgesics twenty-four hours a day, but this creates a problem. The patient may start the drug cycle completely unaware of the end results.

I have found that if a patient complains long enough and loud enough to a physician, pain medication will usually be forthcoming. If the physician refuses, then the patient simply goes to another physician who will write the prescription; or if the dosage is not increased enough, the patient may go to an additional physician, obtain the same prescription and double or even triple the amount of medication taken. Some of these doctor-shopping patients are constantly on the borderline of overdosing themselves. I wish this situation were more the exception, but I'm afraid it's closer to the rule.

But My Doctor Prescribed It!

Pain patients are truly confused when I tell them about the problems of continued use of pain medication. They are bewildered and disbelieving, since their physicians prescribed the medication for them.

Let's take a look at the physician's position. He or she may be in a double bind and could have exhausted all of his or her methods for treating the pain so that analgesics seem to be the only alternative left, other than telling the patient to live with the pain. I know of no state that has a central registry for patients' prescriptions and, therefore, doctors are left without a method of knowing whether a patient is getting a duplicate prescription from another physician and another pharmacy. I have seen people who have as many as four prescriptions for Percodan from four different physicians and obtain the drug from four different pharmacies, with the prescribing physicians totally in the dark.

When these people enter our Pain Control Program, one of the first steps is to coordinate any prescriptions from their physicians. We've talked a lot about analgesics, so let's take a closer look.

The Two Types of Analgesics

Nonnarcotic

There are basically two types of analgesics: nonnarcotic and narcotic. The nonnarcotic analgesics include aspirin and acetaminophen (Tylenol, Datril, Tempra—aspirin substitutes). Since aspirin is nonnarcotic, it can be obtained over the counter and is probably the cheapest and most accessible pain reliever available. After you finish the Pain Control Program, I recommend that aspirin or an aspirin substitute be used until your skills have reached a high enough level to reduce analgesic intake completely.

NOTE: Caffeine, found in coffee, cola and tea, is also considered to be analgesic and may be appropriately used for the relief of some headache conditions. There are also many other nonnarcotic analgesics, which are found in nasal decongestants or cough syrups, all of them providing essentially the same amount of pain relief, but with different combinations of ingredients.

Narcotic

Narcotic pain medications are a completely different story and include: morphine, codeine, Percodan and various other combinations of narcotic ingredients. Narcotics can be prescribed only by a physician and have numerous possible side effects, including addiction. The side effects can override any benefits from the drug's painkilling properties. The previously referred to "drug double bind" can be a direct result of narcotic painkiller abuse.

The Drug Double Bind

Tim L. started out with a mild painkiller, but within eight months he was taking fourteen Percodan a day. His body was accommodated to the medication and only this dosage could provide him enough relief to continue with the day's activities.

No one planned for Tim to become a legalized drug addict, least of all his physician, who had orginally prescribed three Percodan a day. After one month, three Percodan didn't give as much relief, so he went back to the physician, who increased the dosage. This continued on a monthly basis as the medication provided less relief and Tim's physician, at a loss as to what to do, since surgery was not indicated, continued to prescribe higher dosages. Eventually, eight to ten Percodan per day was just enough to get rid of most of the pain, with fourteen leaving him essentially pain-free.

With fourteen per day Tim started to notice personality changes. He would get drowsy or angry and fly off the handle at the least provocation. When he wasn't frustrated or angry, he was depressed. He saw the handwriting on the wall and knew where he was headed. He happened to be a counselor for the Veterans Administration in the alcohol rehabilitation ward. He knew about addiction, both physical and metal, and how alcohol and narcotics were similar in many ways. He was already fast on his way to becoming one of the hundreds of thousands of legalized drug abusers in the United States when I first met him. He was depressed, ready to give up, on the edge of the deep canyon of addiction. The medication was killing him just as surely as if he had placed a gun against the side of his head and pulled the trigger. "I want to get off the stuff," he pleaded, tears filling his eyes, "but nothing else seems to work. The doctor told me I'm going to have to learn to live with the pain, but I can't do my job when I hurt and then how is my family going to survive? I feel like I'm on a merry-go-round and can't get off. Help me, please!"

Tim's situation is a perfect example of the phenomenon known as drug tolerance. He found that even switching to another drug didn't help, since his tolerance seemed to cross over to other medications. (When increased dosages of one drug fail to provide pain relief, many people report that there is a similar reaction to other painkillers.) Tim was a legalized drug addict caught in the double bind of pain medication. We started the Pain Control Program immediately.

With Tim's doctor, I coordinated a program of withdrawal from the narcotic pain medication, and at the same time Tim started achieving success with P.C.P. Imagery. At first it wasn't easy, because withdrawal from drugs isn't easy, but Tim made it! Now he substitutes P.C.P. Imagery for narcotic pain medication. His family, marital and work relationships all improved.

The Withdrawal Reaction

Withdrawal from extended use of narcotic pain medication usually is characterized by certain symptoms that appear in about twenty-four hours. For a few people, these symptoms are minor, but for most, withdrawal is not a pleasant experience. I have compiled a list of common reactions so that you will be aware of some symptoms you could possibly experience while decreasing your medication level. The onset of withdrawal symptoms from reduction of medication usually occurs after one to three days but symptoms may last for up to five or six days. Some of these commonly found withdrawal reactions are listed for you. Transfer the list to your notebook and as your medication is reduced, keep this list in mind.

Withdrawal Symptoms

Restlessness	Chills
Panic	Nausea
The Shakes	Muscle Pain
Rapid Heart Beat	Sweating
Stomach Cramps	Widening of the Pupils
Craving for the Discontinued	of the Eyes
Medication	

> NOTE: Never, under any circumstances, stop taking narcotic medication abruptly. Consult your physician. Abrupt withdrawal from some narcotics can result in very serious side effects. The key word is gradual.

Admitting to Yourself

Probably the most difficult aspect of legalized medication abuse is self-realization that there is a very dangerous situation present that is *not*, in the long run, helping you to solve your pain problem. Addiction is an insidious enemy that sneaks up on you and gradually takes control of your life.

STEP ONE

Admitting you have a problem is possibly the most difficult step. The next step is to list all medications you take for pain, the amount you take, and how frequently you take them. Many people are not aware of the amount they take until they see it listed in black and white. Underneath your list of present medications, list all the previous medications. You may find the list to be a surprisingly failure-ridden history of previous pain control attempts.

Pain Medication

STEP TWO

Here is a questionnaire that will give you an objective reading of your drug dependency. Remember to be totally honest with yourself, since there is no way that I can cross-check any of your answers. As with any of these self-tests, YOU must be your own proctor.

Drug Need Survey

Please read each statement carefully and on a sheet of paper note the number of each question; mark YES or NO beside it as the answer applies to your own particular situation.

1. My physician has increased the strength or amount of my pain medication within the past six months.
2. My physician has prescribed a stronger medication within the past six months.
3. The medication doesn't work as long as it used to.
4. Sometimes I take the medication before the pain gets bad, because I know it's going to be bad.
5. Sometimes I count the pills to make sure I have enough for the weekend.
6. The more I complain, the stronger the medication my doctor gives me.
7. Sometimes I don't know how I'd be able to live without the medication.
8. If I don't have my medication, I become irritable.
9. My doctor has warned me about too much pain medication.
10. I feel that I am too dependent on my pain medication.
11. If my doctor stopped my pain medication, I'd switch doctors.
12. I've tried more than twice to stop taking the medication.

If you have answered YES to any three of the questions, then you may be setting yourself up for legalized drug addiction. You need to find another method of controlling the pain. The Pain Control Program is for YOU.

THERAPY THOUGHT: *Awareness of a potential or existing problem may be the key to prevention.*

STEP THREE

Before you begin your Pain Control Program, call your physician and ask him or her if you can reduce and eventually stop taking your pain medication. He or she will probably tell you to do it gradually. Remember, withdrawal symptoms may be different for each individual and you should constantly refer back to the withdrawal symptom list and check to see if you are experiencing any of these effects.

DO NOT START YOUR WITHDRAWAL FROM PAIN MEDICATION UNTIL YOU HAVE CHECKED WITH YOUR PHYSICIAN AND BEGUN THE P.C.P.

When you start the Pain Control Program in Part II, you will find a Daily Record with spaces for you to record the amount of pain medication you have taken each day. Use this as a guide for the reduction of medication. Since the Pain Control Program lasts two weeks, set fourteen days as your target for being totally free of narcotic pain medications. If your physician agrees, carefully follow the drug reduction rules in the program.

Note: Reducing your medication by no more than 10 percent per day is a good rule of thumb. (However, if you have questions, always consult your physician first.)

5

❧

Anatomy of Pain

Test Your Knowledge!

See how many of these questions you can answer. You may find that you know how pain feels but not *why*. Learning the why of pain is an essential part of the Pain Control Program.

1. What is a nerve cell?
2. How does a synapse affect your pain?
3. How fast do pain impulses travel?
4. How does the autonomic nervous system affect your pain response?
5. What is the difference between sensory and motor neurons?
6. What are the parts of the central nervous system?
7. Why is the peripheral nervous system important?
8. What is the connection between the fight-or-flight response and pain?
9. How do you program yourself for pain?
10. Where do pain engrams start?

If answers to most of these questions eluded you, don't despair, they can all be found within this chapter.

A Short Course in the Nervous System
OR
Everything You've Always Wanted to Know About Nerves but Didn't Know Whom to Ask

A COMPLEX SYSTEM

Most of us are aware of the tremendous complexity of the telephone system and its massive bundles of wires reaching out in every direction from central terminals to individual phones. I have always found it a miracle that a phone call from California can be connected to New York in a short period of time, given the intricacy of the total system. Keep the example of the telephone company in mind and imagine that your body is the total system. Your brain is the central computer (switchboard), which analyzes all the incoming data; the spinal cord (main signal transmission cable) serves as the main relay, which carries transmissions from all parts of the body up to the brain; all of the nerves that go to almost every part of your body resemble telephone wires, and the nerve endings serve as telephones. When you cut yourself or apply cold, heat or an abrasive to the skin, the nerve fibers (telephones) are irritated and send a signal along the pathway, through the spinal cord, to specialized areas of the brain that receive, interpret and classify the message. Where this signal eventually terminates in the brain influences what your next action might be. If the spinal cord is cut or damaged, as happens in some accidents, the messages from the nerves will be blocked at the site of injury and never reach the brain. The lack of messages may create paralysis or, worse, death.

How does the nervous system fit into your pain problem? To learn how the body's built-in painkiller (endorphins) may be activated, you need to understand how pain signals are transported within the body.

THE SPINAL COLUMN: CARRYING NERVE IMPULSES TO AND FROM THE BRAIN

The Nerve Cell

The most basic unit of the nervous system is the nerve cell. Nerve cells are called neurons and are structurally similar to any other cell in the human body. Most neurons consist of a cell body, a long fiber called an axon and several extensions from the other end of the cell body, called dendrites. A nerve may be a single cell or a bundle of cells and can be quite short or as long as several feet. Billions of nerve cells join together to form the nerve networks that serve as the pathways of communication from all parts of the body into the spinal cord and eventually to the brain. In the brain, as the impulses that are sent along the nerve pathway are decoded, we make decisions as to how we should react to any given stimulus. Some of these decisions are conscious while others are unconscious or autonomic (automatic).

A Stimulus-Response System

More than 100 billion nerve cells must work together harmoniously to make one human body work. Reactions to messages received from a multitude of nerve endings are relayed through this stimulus-response system by synaptic connectors, which join one nerve cell to the next.

Synapse—the Connection

It came as quite a shock to researchers when they found that there was a gap between the axon of one nerve cell and the dendrites of the next. The earliest researchers of nervous system activity had assumed that nerve fibers were connected, thus explaining the continuous transmission of nerve impulses. When the gap (synapse) was discovered, scientists postulated that some type of electrical transfer of information took place between the nerve cells. Later they discovered that communication through the synaptic gap is mediated by a chemical transmitter. The substance is released by the ends of the nerve fiber as an impulse arrives. The chemical diffuses into the synaptic gap, facilitating a reaction in the dendrites of the receiving nerve cell. If the receiving nerve cell is excited, the impulse continues on its journey, but if a chemical inhibits the transmission, the nerve impulse will terminate. Literally billions of synaptic responses occur every second of every hour within your body. Synapses serve as the body's internal nerve bridges that transmit pain signals from the site of damage to the brain and back again.

FASTER THAN A SPEEDING BULLET

Not all nerve messages travel at the same speed. The nerve pathways throughout your body are different sizes. The large fibers, known as A-fibers, carry impulses at a very fast speed (15 to 120 meters per second), and the small C-fibers carry impulses between 0.5 and 1.0 meters per second.

A better understanding of the different speeds of nerve impulses can be gained by the following example: while cooking, you reach for a pan on the stove, not realizing that the burner is on low heat. When you touch the pan there is an immediate sensation of pain that causes you to pull your hand away quickly. After a short period of time the pain increases, spreading beyond the part of your hand which touched the hot pan.

What happened? Why the different feelings of pain? The initial pain response was carried by A-fibers, the faster fibers, speeding the signal to the brain the quickest way possible and helping you to pull your hand away from the *dangerous situation.* The secondary C-fibers came into play more slowly than the A-fibers, and this is when you felt the spreading pain. The initial pain response provided by the fastest fibers is necessary to prevent harm to ourselves, but the slower fibers cause the pain to linger after the initial warning signal has been provided.

A Very Impulsive System

I've already mentioned that the nervous system contains several billion neurons, all of which are connected to one another through synapses. Remember, the neurons are nerve cells that pass the information along the nerve network. The dendrites receive the information and pass it through the body of the neuron to the axon, which, through a synapse, passes it to the next dendrite.

All of these actions occur without your being consciously aware of them. We would be in a sorry state if we had to control consciously each synaptic action within the human body. There is no computer presently capable of handling all of the nervous system functions of one individual for one five-minute period. The nervous system is our main life support system and keeps us in touch with everything on the outside and inside.

Windows to the World

All the multitude of nerve endings respond to stimuli within their specific area. Nerve endings may terminate in the skin, eyes, ears, nose or any other part of the body and serve as the brain's information-gathering system. These nerve endings are specialized and tell us whether we are cold or hot, help us to differentiate between different types of smells or tastes; some operate in the internal organs, to help control blood flow, digestion, heart rate, blood pressure and numerous other complicated functions.

Information from the nerve endings is passed on to one of two types of nerve cells (neurons).

- Sensory neurons—neurons that carry sensory information to the spinal cord and to the brain, indicating heat, cold, chemicals, touch, changes in internal organs, light waves, sound waves and any other type of sensory information, including impulses which are interpreted by the brain as pain.

- Motor neurons—neurons that control muscular and glandular functions and help us to walk, run, stand, sit, balance and that assist in the functioning of certain organs.

Putting the Nerves Together

Now that you have a basic understanding of the synapse and neurons, we move on to the total nervous system, which regulates all the activities of the skeletal-muscular system, the digestive system, the respiratory system and the circulatory system. The nervous system is composed of three main divisions:

- The central nervous system (including the brain and spinal cord)
- The peripheral nervous system (the system that extends out from the spinal cord and the base of the brain, and controls various parts of the body)
- The autonomic nervous system (controls and regulates the internal organs)

These divisions work in harmony, keeping all of your body's systems functioning at the optimum. No one expects you to memorize all parts of the system, but to understand how your body works, it is essential that you gain a general overview.

The Central Nervous System

The central nervous system is further divided into five specific areas:

- Cerebrum
- Spinal cord
- Cerebellum
- Pons
- Medulla oblongata

Each area of the brain has its own specific function; arriving signals activate our response mechanisms, such as pupil dilation, moving an arm or leg, breathing deeper or controlling some internal organ.

SUMMARY OF THE CENTRAL NERVOUS SYSTEM

The central nervous system is made up of the brain and spinal cord. The brain is the centralized computer for controlling all functions including thoughts, reasoning and judgment. Your skull protects your brain. Your spinal cord is protected by your backbone. Each bone in the spinal column has an opening through which the spinal cord passes. As a further protection, cerebral-spinal fluid is contained within a sac that closely surrounds the spinal cord and brain. The fluid serves as a shock absorber for any jarring of the brain or spinal cord. The spinal cord is made up of nerve tissue and is a direct continuation of the brain. It serves as the main connection link between the peripheral nervous system (peripheral meaning away from the center or out to the side) and the brain. All nerve impulses and messages must pass through the spinal cord in order to reach the brain.

The central nervous system keeps you functioning whether you are at work or deep in sleep, day and night.

The Peripheral Nervous System

The peripheral nervous system is composed of nerve structures outside of the brain and the spinal cord and connects the central nervous system with the periphery of the body. This peripheral system includes twelve pairs of cranial nerves and thirty-one pairs of spinal nerves.

The twelve pairs of cranial nerves, which exit through the base of the skull, control such functions as smell, vision, eye movements, mastication (chewing), taste, muscle sense, hearing, sense of balance, swallowing, cutaneous sensations of the ear, hunger, pain, respiratory reflexes, movements of the neck, shoulder and soft palate, and muscular movements of the tongue. These cranial nerves also affect many other areas because of their complex network of nerve fibers.

The thirty-one pairs of spinal nerves, arising from the spinal cord, are composed of the following pairs: eight cervical, twelve thoracic, five lumbar, five sacral, one coccygeal. Each of these nerves is attached to the spinal cord by two roots (anterior and posterior), which unite a short distance away from the cord. Each of these nerve roots branches out into various parts of the body, whether into the chest or down to the legs, controlling all functions.

Whenever there is damage to the spinal cord, functions controlled by nerves below the level of the injury are not carried out. Nerves that emanate from the spinal cord into other areas also explain why some people with back injuries experience referred pain in such areas as the leg, foot and thigh.

Understanding the functions of the peripheral nervous system can help you move into the realm of the autonomic nervous system.

The Autonomic Nervous System

The autonomic nervous system regulates the activities of numerous organs not usually under our conscious control. Such organs as the heart function continuously without continual, conscious thought. If the operation of your heart were totally under your conscious control, you could become distracted while simply concentrating on talking with another person and die from lack of a message to the heart muscle. There is an obvious need for automatic functioning of some parts of the body. But do we have any control over the autonomic nervous system?

Only during the last decade have researchers found that the autonomic nervous system *can* be controlled, in part, through conscious training. Some Eastern religions gave us the first clues through amazing feats of body control, such as slowing or stopping the heartbeat, controlling bleeding and pain.

Our emotions directly influence the functions of the autonomic nervous system. The inborn fight-or-flight response is a good example of a split-second autonomic reaction.

Fight or Flight
The fight-or-flight response is an inborn response exhibited by every human. This bodily reaction occurs so quickly that within a split second numerous body functions are affected. Take an example:

You're staying overnight in a strange town, and at eleven o'clock in the evening you decide to go out to buy a magazine. The street is very dark and deserted, bathed in the eerie shadows of street lights. Halfway to the store, you pass an alleyway and suddenly a figure leaps out at you.

The actions of the figure from the shadows take place in a matter of seconds. But something even faster has happened within your body, automatically!

First, the hypothalamus (part of your brain) chemically signals the pituitary gland, which in turn sends ACTH hormone to the adrenal glands resting above the kidneys. The outer layer, or cortex, of each adrenal gland secretes cortical steroids, which flow through the gland's inner core, or medulla, and set off an immediate outpouring of adrenaline into your circulating bloodstream. As this happens, the blood vessels of the skin contract and blood is forced away from the extremities and into the muscles of the vital organs. Your heartbeat increases, and there is a rise in blood pressure. Simultaneously, adrenaline in the liver chemically converts stored glycogen into active blood sugar (glucose) for fueling nerve and muscle cells with extra energy. At the same time, still more adrenaline dilates the bronchi in the lungs to allow a maximum intake of oxygen; dilates the pupils of the eyes (the startled response); contracts the spleen, forcing out its reserve supply of red blood cells; activates chemicals that speed up coagulation of the blood in the event of injury; and increases the tension of voluntary muscles.

All of the reactions that occur during the fight-or-flight response are activated in a split second. Can you imagine trying to control them by conscious thought? A good understanding of the fight-or-flight response will prepare you for learning to activate your own built-in painkillers through Pain Control Imagery (P.C.I.).

Programing the System

Like a computer, the human nervous system is constantly obtaining various types of information, which is evaluated, stored and processed. Much in the same way as a computer, we program our responses in the brain by habit formation (repetition). Whenever an event occurs, the program is activated and we react as we did in the past when presented with like circumstances. All of our pain experiences are programed into our brain's response mechanisms. When you stub your toe and the pain signal reaches your brain, it is as if a switch were thrown and the program for your pain response begins. These programs in your brain are known as engrams.

Any time you experience pain, an engram is imprinted within the body's nervous system and brain. This printed circuit is embossed into your pattern of pain perception, and even when the injury, stress or disease is eliminated, the engram of pain may remain until reprogramed. Engrams are resistant to change unless a systematic reprograming effort is initiated.

When you constantly think about pain and suffering, you are reinforcing the pain engrams within your system. Pain engrams can be like a needle stuck on a record, and important body functions will take a back seat to the repeated pain program.

Each and every time you suffer from pain, this experience is recorded within the memory banks of your brain in much the same way as you record something on a tape recorder. At a later date, possibly under the same circumstances, the memory is recalled and you may feel the pain even before there is any injury to the body. In other words, the memory of old pain and anticipation of new can actually bring about the pain response.

Someone who has burned a finger on a hot stove can experience similar pain long after the initial injury is healed whenever his hand is placed near a burner, even if the stove is off. Your thought processes anticipate the pain and activate the pain engram, which can produce pain although there is no injury to the body. The beginnings of pain engrams usually can be found in a person's childhood.

Childhood—the First Step in Programing

Examination of the development of pain engrams leads us to the conclusion that a large part of the pain response is learned. Pain may be lessened by a systematic reprograming of our pain response behavior.

The environment in which we grow up has a direct effect upon our perception of and reaction to pain. Dr. Ronald Melzak, pain researcher at McGill University, demonstrated learned pain response through an experiment with a group of

Scottie dogs raised in a totally restricted environment. From infancy to maturity, they had no opportunity to exchange and learn the rules of proper social interaction among other dogs or humans. They were totally isolated during their first months of development. Melzak was amazed to find that the dogs had not developed normal pain sensitivity. They seemed to have no sense of pain, or at least nothing more than a brief reflex response to a harmful stimulus. They would return again and again to a burning match until it severely burned their nose. His dogs would explore the burning match a second time, as if they were not burned the first time. These experiments have been duplicated with chimpanzees raised in a similar restricted environment. Therefore, it seems logical to assume that reaction to pain (pain engrams) may be a process partially developed through socialization (a learned reaction).

The Pain Control Program is specifically designed to teach you how to reprogram your pain engrams by learning to control present pain and prevent future pain.

Future Pain

Understanding the dynamics of pain engrams can serve as a first step in the reduction of pain. If a doctor who is about to inject you says, "Slight pinprick," this may help you feel only a slight pinprick. But if that same doctor says, "This is going to hurt," then there is a good chance that a pain engram may click in automatically, causing an increase in your discomfort.

Pain, arising from fear of and anxiety about the unknown, confronts dentists daily. The whistling, grinding sound of the drill, the thought of injections into the soft tissues of the mouth, the sudden stab of pain as an unprotected nerve is accidentally jabbed, are uppermost in the minds of most patients as they sit in the waiting room building up their anticipation of discomfort before receiving treatment. Whenever I speak before a group of dentists, I find them concerned with how to reduce the patient's fear of future pain. Some of the suggestions I give them to help their patients can help you. Whenever you start to anticipate pain, try these simple steps:

Step One: Find out what's going to happen. Don't allow yourself to remain in the dark; that's when fears build. Ask questions and be willing to hear the answers.

Step Two: Use methods such as pain thought stopping to terminate your thoughts of future pain. (See Chapter Sixteen.)

Step Three: Don't exhibit pain reactions just because you think you're going to be in pain, for this can activate a pain engram.

Step Four: Use the two pain control techniques outlined in Chapter Two to prevent yourself from pumping up the pain.

Moving On

We now are ready to learn about foods and how they affect pain and YOU!

6

֎§§֎

How Food Can Feed Your Pain

Very few aspects of daily living have received as much attention as diet. Almost invariably, a new diet develops weekly and millions of Americans madly rush to find the miracle cure for weight loss. While most chase vainly after the elusive butterfly of weight loss, diet is directly related to another, and possibly just as devastating, problem in our lives. I'm talking about the relationship between what you eat and pain.

Diet directly affects various types of pain, the most prominent being headache. Knowledge and avoidance of those substances that have been known to increase pain may save you from long hours of suffering.

Right now is the time to eliminate systematically many of these probable causes of pain from your diet.

THERAPY THOUGHT: *Always check with your physician before drastically altering your diet.*

The Painful Six

Any discussion of food and its relationship to pain, especially headache, should take into consideration the fact that medical schools have only recently introduced dietary instruction into the medical curriculum. Many medical schools still do not consider an individual's food intake to be relevant to the pain problem. But there is evidence to show that some headaches are directly caused by diet.

Dr. Ellen C. G. Grant, at Charing Cross Hospital in London, has been studying systematic elimination of high risk food. Dr. Grant and her researchers began by stopping oral contraceptives, smoking and ergotamine medication (used to treat migraine). Eliminating these substances helped many people but the study expanded to sixty migraine patients who were found to have migraine reactions to an average of ten foods each. The most common "migraine" foods are wheat, oranges, eggs, tea and coffee, chocolate, milk, beef, corn, cane sugar and yeast.

When contraindicated foods are identified and eliminated from the diet, a substantial reduction of pain, especially that of the headache, follows.

Let's take a look at what parts of your diet could lead to pain.

MONOSODIUM GLUTAMATE (MSG)

Dr. James W. Lane, an Australian neurologist, was the first to describe the "Chinese restaurant syndrome." He found that within twenty to thirty minutes after eating Chinese food some people develop a variety of unpleasant symptoms, which include headache, sweating, pounding pain over the temples and a tightness around the forehead. At first, he thought it might be some type of contamination. After exhaustive research, the food additive and flavor enhancer monosodium glutamate (MSG) was found to be the culprit. The only way to detect whether you are sensitive to MSG is to determine whether you have any of these symptoms after eating Chinese food. MSG is one of the major ingredients in won ton soup, usually served at the beginning of a meal when your stomach is empty, which makes the effect of MSG even more dramatic.

Some researchers estimate that 10 to 15 percent of the population may be sensitive to MSG. If you are sensitive to this food additive, you may not experience all of the symptoms and the headache may be the only one you recognize.

The immediate answer seems quite simple. Avoid eating Chinese food. But the solution is not totally uncomplicated, for the flavor-enhancing ability of MSG causes it to be used in the processing of some non-Chinese foods.

Monosodium glutamate may be found in many different items, including Accent and other tenderizers, and in some, but not all

Frozen dinners	Ham and bacon
Self-basting turkeys	Soy sauce
Dry-roasted nuts	Processed meats
Instant gravies	Instant soups
Canned soups	

Read the Label

There is one sure way to avoid MSG in your diet if headache is a problem for you, and that is to read labels carefully. If you notice that MSG is one of the ingredients, then avoid that food and you may be taking away one of the causes of your headache. Foods containing MSG are not vital to our survival and can be replaced with alternative foods.

NITRITES

Have you ever suffered a headache after eating any of the following:

Hot dogs	Bacon
Ham	Sausage
Smoked fish	Corned beef
Salami	Canned hams
Bologna	

If so, you might suffer from the "hot dog headache." Almost all of these foods contain nitrates and nitrites, which are used as a preservative to cure meats. At the present time the Federal Drug Administration is investigating the possibility that nitrates and nitrites might be carcinogenic (cancer producing), but regulations regarding the use of these chemicals seem to be mired in political lobbying and contested test results in animals.

Why do nitrite compounds cause headaches? These substances cause your blood vessels to dilate, creating the pounding, vascular type of headache in those who are vulnerable. Nitrite compounds are a derivative of nitroglycerin, which is used to ease the effects of heart attacks and angina pain. For many years, workers who handled dynamite knew that nitrites absorbed through the skin could induce headaches.

I had a patient who told me that barbecuing hot dogs on an outdoor grill removed all of the nitrites. I had another tell me that boiling them would also remove nitrites. Dietary scientists whom I've consulted advise that neither method is effective in removing nitrites and the only true way to remove this substance from your diet is to avoid eating foods containing it.

Elimination of nitrites and nitrates from your diet would help reduce your discomfort. Copy the nitrite list into your pain notebook. Give it a try. We all can do without hot dogs, bacon and some processed foods for a while.

CAFFEINE

Dan was a heavy coffee drinker, consuming daily twelve to fifteen cups of coffee, two to three soft drinks and occasionally some chocolate. During the day, he noticed an increase in his nervousness, and sometimes at night he would have trouble sleeping. He almost always had a headache when awakening, and then later on in the day, the headache would return. His physician referred him to me. During the course of our discussion I asked him about his caffeine intake. I suggested he discontinue his coffee, cola, chocolate and any other caffeine-containing substances to see if that helped relieve his headache. Within two weeks nearly all of the anxiety symptoms and the headaches had stopped. But how had caffeine caused Dan's headaches, especially on waking in the morning, when obviously he had not been drinking coffee?

Caffeine constricts the blood vessels, making them smaller, and this narrowing of the blood vessels limits the flow of blood through the body. Caffeine also acts as a stimulant to the heart and brain and has been know to raise the blood sugar level, stimulate urine production and increase the assimilation of some medications. During the day, Dan would ingest tremendous amounts of caffeine and develop a caffeine headache toward the latter part of the day. During the evening hours, he reduced his caffeine intake; by early morning the blood vessels had dilated (expanded) and this led to what is known as a rebound headache. The only way for Dan to get out of such a vicious cycle was to eliminate his intake of caffeine completely.

Eliminating caffeine from your diet may be harder than you think. Take a look at this partial list that contain caffeine. How many do you take daily?

Coffee	Chocolate drinks
Tea	Medications such as Excedrin,
Cola	Vanquish, Empirin, most
Chocolate	sinus headache drugs and
Instant coffee	cold capsules

So the next time you want to take a coffee break, turn it into a pain break and try eliminating caffeine completely from your diet. When you take yourself off caffeine products, be aware that you might suffer the effects of a rebound headache initially, but this will disappear after your body readjusts to life without caffeine.

THERAPY THOUGHT: *The only way to determine definitely whether caffeine is a contributing factor to your headaches is to eliminate caffeine totally from your diet.*

ALCOHOL

If you suffer from headaches, particularly the vascular type of headache, try eliminating alcohol totally. Alcohol expands blood vessels and may bring about throbbing, vascular discomfort. Alcohol rebound headaches are sometimes confused with hangovers. Recent research by allergists indicates that women may be more susceptible to the artificial chemicals that provide flavor or coloring in some alcoholic drinks. These artificial ingredients could also contribute to your pain. If you must drink, vodka is probably the safest alcoholic beverage, since it contains the fewest additives.

Alcoholic drinks such as beer and wine contain a wide variety of ingredients from corn to grapes, and if you are allergic to any of these, headaches may be just around the corner. As with other dietary considerations that affect a pain problem, the best way to determine alcohol's effect is to eliminate it totally. By doing so you may also reduce the risk of other physical problems associated with alcohol.

NICOTINE HEADACHES

Susan always developed a headache when she was in a room filled with smokers. When she left the smoke-filled room, the headache pain would lessen.

The effect of nicotine on Susan's blood vessels was to constrict them (make them smaller). This was serving as a headache trigger and was a direct cause of her discomfort.

If you are a smoker and develop headaches after smoking for a period of time, you may also suffer from nicotine headache rebound, which is essentially the same as the caffeine or alcohol rebound headache. Many people who are heavy smokers find that they awaken in the morning with a headache, but after the first cigarette the pain lessens (the nicotine has constricted the blood vessels). But as the day progresses, they develop the true nicotine headache.

The only way off the nicotine pain merry-go-round is to quit smoking totally and see if this eliminates your discomfort.

TYRAMINE

No discussion of dietary implications in pain would be complete without tyramine. This chemical dilates blood vessels and may be a contributing or leading factor in some headache problems. Tyramine is mostly found in aged cheeses, red wines, some meat and fish, and assorted dairy products. As with other elements just mentioned, the only way to check your sensitivity to tyramine is careful avoidance of the products that contain it.

. . . It Isn't Easy

In this chapter I have listed many substances that could contribute to your pain problems, particularly headaches. There is no one simple answer as to which might affect you in particular.

The only test is to totally eliminate from your diet those that might cause your headaches and to record carefully the effect of their elimination. This could mean giving up some favorite foods, but ask yourself if one throbbing, pulsating headache is worth five cups of coffee.

You may be surprised at the pain reduction that occurs when you pay close attention to what you eat, drink or take into your body.

7

◆§❦◆

A Mini Dictionary of Pain

Knowledge about the various types of pain and their causes can be very helpful in any search for the answer to chronic pain. The descriptions and causes of various pain problems that follow are in no way meant to replace proper medical diagnosis.

ARTERIOSCLEROSIS

This type of pain may be caused by increased build-up of fat deposits, which may be a direct result of a high-cholesterol diet, inactivity or inherited characteristics.

ARTHRITIS

The Facts
- Arthritis is the nation's number-one crippler.
- Arthritis affects close to 40 million Americans.
- Arthritis is the most costly disease in the United States, with a total economic impact, including lost wages and medical bills, of $14 billion a year.
- Since most people don't die of arthritis, the suffering may be long and devastating.

Types of Arthritis
There are over 100 separate and distinct diseases of the joints and connective tissues that are generally classified as arthritis.

71

To simplify matters, arthritis has been divided into two general categories:

Rheumatoid arthritis: an inflammation of the soft tissues of the joint lining that causes hot, swollen joints, fatigue and often fever. In some stages it can affect the heart, lungs and other organ systems. Children may be affected with juvenile rheumatoid arthritis (JRA).

Osteoarthritis: This type of arthritis is frequently referred to as the degenerative arthritis. It is focused mostly on the joints and eventually erodes the cartilage in the joint areas, leading to immobility.

Cause of Pain

In arthritis there is inflammation of joints, impairment of movement. There may be some bone and joint deterioration. In acute phases, arthritis is marked by pain, heat, redness, and swelling due to inflammation, infection or trauma.

ANGINA PAIN

Angina pain has been variously described as spasmlike, choking or suffocating pain. This type of pain is almost always associated with angina pectoris. Many times this pain may be caused by effort or excitement. Some people experiencing this pain for the first time become quite scared and fear impending death. Part of the pain may be due to a lack of oxygen to certain parts of the heart (myocardium). In some cases the condition may be fatal.

BUERGER'S DISEASE

This disease is typically found in young males and appears to have a characteristic location and a very definite set of symptoms. Buerger's disease affects the small arteries of the feet and hands and there is usually intense inflammation and accompanying severe pain.

The use of Pain Control Imagery may increase blood flow to the extremities, especially the hands, and thereby increase warmth and reduce the pain.

BURSITIS

The fluid-filled sacs that surround the joints are known as bursae. When they become inflamed, a condition known as bursitis may evolve. Injury, infection or strain may be causes of bursitis; tennis elbow and floor cleaner's knee are examples.

CANCER PAIN

Sometimes for the cancer victim, death serves as the only escape from the intolerable sensations of blockage of organs and destruction of bones and tissues by tumors and the effect of tumor growth on sensitive nerves. Radiation and chemotherapy may also produce severe iatrogenic (treatment-caused) pain, which can add to an already overburdened nervous system.

CAUSALGIA (REFLEX SYMPATHETIC DYSTROPHY)

The causes of this pain include trauma, surgery, repeated abuse, infection, myocardial infarction (heart attack), and vascular disorders. This syndrome is characterized by a constant, severe burning pain which may continue even after the injury has healed. The apparent cause of this pain is nerve damage, which may take years to heal.

FOOT AND ANKLE PAIN

These types of pain may be caused by rheumatoid arthritis, osteoarthritis, gout, tendonitis, flat feet, hammertoe or bruised heel pad. With the national interest in running, there has been a large increase in the number of people experiencing foot and ankle pain.

GOUT

Technically, gout is a build-up of uric acid in various body joints. Under normal circumstances uric acid is produced by the kidneys and eliminated through the urine, but when there has been damage to the kidneys, the acid may find its way into very sensitive joints. Anyone suffering from gout should be under the close supervision of a physician who specializes in this type of disorder.

HEADACHES

There are numerous types of headaches, including muscle contraction headaches, cluster headaches and migraine headaches. These headaches may arise from many different sources, such as tension, diet, blood vessel abnormalities, trauma to the head, neck injuries and numerous types of tumors. For a more concise look at headaches, please refer to Chapter Eight.

HERPES ZOSTER (SHINGLES)

The same virus that causes chicken pox in youngsters may lead to this painful condition. Lesions may form on the surface of the skin and under the skin which directly affect the nerve endings. Large amounts of damage may be caused to nerve fibers (post-herpetic neuralgia) and pain is usually intensive and may continue for long periods of time.

HIP PAIN

This type of pain is most commonly associated with osteo-arthritis in older people. Bursitis of the thigh may also cause this pain.

ICE-CREAM HEADACHES

Take a warm summer day and an ice-cold drink or ice-cream cone and you have all the ingredients for an ice-cream headache. When the blood vessels in the palate (upper roof of the mouth) come in contact with cool substances, the blood vessels constrict, cutting off the flow of blood to the sinuses, regions of the eye (ophthalmic arteries) and forehead. Eating and drinking more slowly and allowing the palate to warm usually erases the headache rapidly.

LOW BACK PAIN

Low back pain may be generated by damage to muscles, ligaments or discs. Sometimes we find a combination of causes for low back pain. This pain may radiate down the legs and is considered one of the major pain problems. For more information, please refer to Chapter Nine.

DIABETIC NEURITIS

For many people suffering from diabetes, a pins-and-needles sensation develops, combined with pain, in the feet and toes. This condition may become quite severe and is usually caused by nerve damage from the diabetes.

NECK PAIN

There are a number of possible causes for neck pain, including poor posture, arthritis, injury, and degeneration of discs between the neck vertebrae called spondylosis which could lead to a slipping of one vertebra forward on the one below causing a condition known as spondylolisthesis. This condition can occur in other regions of the back as well as in the neck.

NEUROMAS

This type of chronic pain may be caused by tumors that develop on nerve endings. If a nerve has been damaged or cut during an accident, neuromas may form, which in turn cause a lasting and, in most cases, untreatable pain.

PHANTOM LIMB PAIN

Many people who have suffered an amputation of one of their limbs report the sensation of pain in the limb that was amputated. This pain may also arise out of improperly healed scars and nerve damage from surgery. In many cases, the pain is generated psychologically and can be devastating.

PALATAL MYOCLONUS

This type of pain may be set off by a neurological disorder or vascular disease centered in the area of the brain stem. Defining the exact area may be difficult in many cases, but the general location of pain is quite clear. Most of the discomfort comes from the palate or roof of the mouth and is caused by quick expansion and contraction of muscles in that area. Muscles of the neck, face and head may also be involved with palatal myoclonus.

POSTOPERATIVE PAIN

After most surgery there is pain that disappears after a normal period of time. If this pain continues after the normal healing processes have taken place, it is known as postoperative pain. In many cases this pain is a type of causalgia or neuralgia which may have resulted from unintentional damage to a nerve during the surgical process. Sometimes there is muscle damage, which may take a longer period of time to heal. Also, the pain could be of psychological origin.

RAYNAUD'S DISEASE

This is a circulatory disease most prevalent in the hands. Because of spasms of the arteries, the blood flow is reduced, which causes an increase in pain and may lead to such serious complications as gangrene.

SCIATICA

This pain is found along the sciatic nerve in the leg. It can come from a herniated disc or muscle spasm in the lower back, which causes pressure to be placed on the sciatic nerve and results in pain down the leg.

STOMACH PAIN

Stomach and intestinal pain may be caused by heartburn, gallstones, chronic constipation, ulcers, ileitis, colitis, hepatitis, pancreatitis, cancer, diverticulitis, diarrhea, gas pains, hemorrhoids and the common stomach ache. Some forms of chronic stomach pain are directly tied to emotions such as stress, anxiety and tension.

Some causes of stomach pain may be improper diet, overdoses of laxatives, too much aspirin, overuse of alcohol, overuse of coffee or beverages containing caffeine, stress and inability to handle unpleasant situations.

TENNIS ELBOW

This is a strain of the muscle over the outer side of the elbow. The bony point at the side of the elbow is tender and pain may radiate down to fingers. Tennis players may develop this condition with improper backhand strokes, but people in occupations that require extensive use of the arm are also susceptible to the condition.

TENDONITIS

When tendons become inflamed we have a condition known as tendonitis. The tendon connects various muscles to the bone. For example, the biceps muscle in the upper arm is joined to the shoulder by a large tendon that, when inflamed, causes biceps tendonitis. Tendonitis causes pain most commonly in the shoulder.

TRIGEMINAL NEURALGIA

This is an irritation of the fifth cranial nerve that may cause facial pain so severe that it is totally disabling. Another name for this pain is tic douloureux.

When to See Your Doctor

Pain is a warning signal that something is wrong with your body; it may be accompanied by other descriptive symptoms. But how do you know when to see the doctor?

I have developed the following checklists to help you determine when to see a doctor for pain and/or accompanying symptoms. Copy the lists into your notebook. They're important!

The Symptom Checklists

If you have any of the symptoms listed for a particular pain, your doctor should be contacted immediately.

STOMACH PAIN

1. Pain that is very severe.
2. Pain that is steady, lasting more than six hours.
3. Pain that is recurring and unexplained.
4. Pain that is accompanied by chills and cold clammy skin.
5. Bowel movements that are sudden, or a persistent change in bowel habits. Bowel movements containing blood, pus or mucus in the stool.
6. Bowel movements that contain black, tarry stools.
7. Bowel movements that contain gray or clay-colored stools.
8. Fever that is persistent for more than two days. Fever that is unexplained and recurring and greater than 101°F.
9. Constant loss of appetite or unintentional weight loss.
10. Pain encountered in swallowing food.

NOTE: Children experiencing stomach pain that lasts more than one or two hours and is accompanied by loss of appetite, vomiting or fever, should be seen by a doctor immediately.

ARTHRITIS AND RHEUMATISM PAIN

1. Morning stiffness lasting more than an hour.
2. Inability to do normal activities.
3. Severe pain at night causing loss of sleep or awakening you.
4. Severe pain in or near joints.
5. Swelling of a joint or joints.
6. Redness of the skin over the joint or joints.
7. Excessive tenderness when you press on a joint.
8. Joint pains lasting more than a week.
9. Swelling and pain that moves from one joint to the next.
10. Restriction in limb movement.
11. Any one of the following:

Rash	Hair loss
Loss of appetite	Diarrhea
Muscle weakness	Tingling
Pins-and-needles in toes or fingers	Loss of weight
	Change of color of fingers or toes when cold

NOTE: Some common infections such as colds, flu or viruses may cause muscular or joint pain. These pains usually disappear after several days and should not be confused with more severe pains that last for a longer period of time.

HEADACHES

1. When you are frequently awakened in the morning by headache pain.
2. Sudden and unexpected vomiting that is not associated with nausea (projectile vomiting).
3. Vision that goes to gray or black for a few seconds and is repeated several times (obscuration).
4. Becoming sleepy or drowsy during the headache.
5. Severe headache pain when in a particular posture.
6. Being awakened from a sound sleep by headache pain.
7. Aches that are initiated by coughing or straining.
8. Headache pain associated with a recent head injury.
9. Numbness or tingling in arms, fingers or one side of the body.
10. Any types of seizures associated with your headache pain.
11. A stiff neck that comes on suddenly with headache pain.
12. Any headache that lasts for more than two to four hours and is not relieved by aspirin or other over-the-counter medications.

BACK PAIN

1. If the pain is new and sudden.
2. Pain accompanied by tingling, then numbness in one or both legs.
3. Pain that awakens you from a sound sleep.
4. Numbness and tingling in the arms and fingers.
5. Shooting pains down the back of the leg.
6. Any back pain that lasts more than two days and is not resolved through bed rest, ice packs and mild analgesics such as aspirin.

NOTE: Pain in the back may involve other systems of the body and you may be referred to a specialist such as a gastroenterologist, urologist, gynecologist, vascular surgeon or neuro-surgeon.

CHEST PAIN

1. Pressure pain or feeling of tightness in the chest.
2. A feeling as if a band is being tightened around the chest.
3. Chest pain that lessens when you sit up.
4. Pain that is felt in the center of the chest under the breast-bone.
5. Pain that is slightly to the left side of the chest and may extend to one or both arms.
6. Pain that moves along the inside of the arm.
7. A heavy or numb feeling in the arm associated with the chest pain.
8. Pain in the throat or jaw associated with chest pain.
9. Pain that lasts between one minute and five minutes, or longer.
10. Pain that worsens on a deep breath.
11. Chest pain that is brought on by physical or emotional stress.
12. Drastic change in any pattern of chest pain.
13. Pain accompanied by sweating, nausea, light-headedness, limb weakness or a change in skin color.

NOTE: Any change in chest pain or development of the above symptoms should be reported to a doctor *immediately*.

KIDNEY AND URINARY PAIN

1. Pain felt during urination (urethral pain). This pain may continue after urination is stopped.
2. Pain felt only during urination (bladder pain) followed by a dull ache or sensation of pressure in the lower abdomen.
3. Constant, very severe pain (urethral pain) may signify the passage of a kidney stone.
4. Pain felt in the back just below the lowest rib that is dull and aching and increased by pressure on that area (kidney pain).
5. Blood in the urine.

6. Difficulty in urination (possible sign of bladder irritation).

7. Incontinence (involuntary urination).

8. Unexplained fever accompanying kidney or urinary pain.

9. Kidney or urinary pain accompanied by swollen ankles.

NOTE: Kidney pain may often be accompanied by fever.

8

✑§§∂✑

Headache:
The Most Common Pain

Julius Caesar	Thomas Jefferson
John Calvin	Sigmund Freud
Miguel de Cervantes	Kareem Abdul-Jabbar
Karl Marx	Ulysses S. Grant
Lewis Carroll	Peter Ilyich Tchaikowsky
Charles Darwin	George Bernard Shaw
Frédéric Chopin	Edgar Allan Poe
Virginia Woolf	

What do all these people and many more have in common? They are all headache sufferers. It has been estimated that over 94 percent of all headaches are benign (not caused by physical defects). The latest studies show that more than half of all doctor visits are for headache-related problems. An estimated 46 million people in the United States alone suffer from chronic headaches. One study showed that ten thousand aspirins are swallowed each minute in New York City, and most are for headaches. National statistics also show that over 80 percent of all headache sufferers are women.

The facts and figures are staggering when you consider the amount of time and money spent for headache medications, both prescription and nonprescription. Headaches are big business in the United States, and if you doubt this, just listen to the radio, watch television or open any magazine and review the staggering numbers of ads for pain relievers.

It's amazing to realize that over 60 percent of people who suffer from headaches do not seek treatment by physicians. They are self-treated through over-the-counter medications and unproven treatments.

A Short History of Headache Treatment

The history of headache treatment is long and involved, reaching as far back as prehistoric times. Here are some of the more interesting treatments.

A. Possibly the first surgical procedure was for headache relief. Early man tried to relieve the pain of headaches by cutting circular holes into the skull. This procedure was known as trepanning. Early people evidently viewed the holes as an escape hatch for "evil spirits," pressures or other influences possibly of a religious nature. Famous trepanning skulls, found along the shores of Lake Titicaca, date back to pre-Columbian Incas of Peru. Amazingly, trepanning is still being practiced by some primitive people of the South Pacific, the Caucasus and Algeria.

B. Probably the earliest descriptive treatment of headache comes from one of the two oldest medical books in existence, the Ebers Papyrus. Discovered in an ancient Egyptian tomb in Thebes, it contains over 900 medical prescriptions, many of them for "a sickness of half the head."

C. Attaching leeches to the body to induce bleeding, an attempted relief of migraine headaches.

D. Application or ingestion of such substances as cow's brain, goat dung, beaver testes bottled in spirits, peppermint, opium, mercury, ammonia—and even hanging a dead buzzard from the neck of the sufferer.

E. Peandius Dioscorides, a surgeon in Nero's army, suggested the use of the torpedo fish (ray) to produce an electrical shock for the cure of headache pain.

We seem to have come a long way from the torpedo fish and the hole in the head, but have we? Headache still plagues us day in and day out and thousands of people still hope for miracle cures. Down through the centuries all of our efforts have been directed toward a cure from outside of the body. Finally, we are looking inward, toward the body's own painkiller, endorphin, for the ultimate answer to headache. The Pain Control Program will provide you with the skills to call on this substance and put an end to headache suffering.

Starting with a Definition

It is easy to see why the word "headache" has been used as an overall term to describe a wide variety of pain problems involving the head, neck and even the shoulders. A statement by the late Dr. H. G. Wolff, professor of neurology at Cornell University Medical School, really summed it up.

Since the human animal prides himself on "using his head," it is ironic and perhaps not without meaning that his head should be the source of so much discomfort. Though pain always means "something wrong," with headache it most often means "wrong direction" or "wrong pace"—a biological reprimand rather than a threat. Thus, the vast majority of discomforts and pains of the head stem from readily reversible bodily changes, and are accompaniments of resentments and dissatisfactions.

Types of Headache

TENSION HEADACHE

The tension headache is probably the most prevalent pain felt by the widest variety of people. Tension headaches have been known as the muscle contraction headache, defensive headache or nervous tension headache. They may be the longest lasting of all headaches, often present for weeks, months or even years.

Cause: As the name implies, tension headaches are caused mostly by muscular contraction, and this in turn may be a direct result of emotional tension and stress. Tensing of the large muscles of the shoulder, which run up to the back of the head, or tensing the muscles covering the skull and face, is a defensive reaction to stress, anxiety or discomfort. Prolonged tension causes sustained contraction of the neck and head muscles and constriction of the small arteries in the scalp and face. Nerve impulses pass to the central nervous system and are sent to the brain, where they are interpreted as pain.

The tensing of muscles is usually an automatic response and until recently was not thought to be in our control. The most effective medications for tension headache have been analgesic substances that dull the sensation of pain and sedate the individual, who then becomes relaxed and thereby decreases the muscular tension and breaks the headache cycle.

Incidence: Dr. Janet Travell, the late President John F. Kennedy's personal physician, feels that 90 percent of all headaches are tension (mechanical) headaches. It is also interesting to note that over 40 percent of tension headache sufferers have a family history of this affliction.

Why They Hurt: The constant muscular contraction of the tension headache causes the blood vessels to become constricted and reduces the flow of blood and prevents the fatigued muscle from becoming renourished. Usually the muscles of the shoulders, neck and scalp are sensitive to touch. The tension headache can also drain a large portion of your energy.

What Do Tension Headaches Feel Like?

- "It feels like a band around my head."
- "My whole face hurts."
- "It feels like someone squeezing my head."
- "It comes without any warning."
- "It feels as though the top of my head had been blown off."
- "Pain is all over my head."
- "The pain seems to be on both sides of my head."
- "It feels like I'm wearing a hat that's too small."
- "My jaws and neck seem to ache."
- "It's a dull, throbbing ache."

- "It feels like someone's pressing against the back of my head."
- "The pain makes me feel dizzy."
- "It hurts when I think."

Do any of these sound familiar?

CASE

Kathy knew what headaches were! She'd been suffering from them, off and on, for the past twelve years. As a secretary and then as a wife and mother, she had experienced the nagging, throbbing pain of tension headaches. The discomfort would grow from the back of her shoulders and make its way up the sides of her neck and across the top of her head. Gradually, the suffering became a way of life. Some mornings she would wake up after what was a good night's sleep and the headache would be there, but most of the time it occurred in the afternoon. She suffered from feelings of inadequacy, guilt and loneliness. The headaches were affecting every aspect of her life, even her sexual relationship with her husband.

It was hard for Kathy to believe that the headaches were directly related to her emotions. The diagnosis of tension headache had been made by seven doctors to whom she had gone. One physician referred her to a psychiatrist, but after six months of analysis little had changed. Day after day, she tried to live with the headaches. What had started during her senior year of high school as an isolated throbbing in the back of her neck was now a chronic affliction.

CHECKLIST FOR TENSION HEADACHES

Seldom are tension headaches caused by only one specific problem; rather, they involve a combination of actions. Carefully read through the following symptoms and record in your notebook *any* that apply to your particular situation:

(NOTE: This checklist is not meant to serve as a substitute for medical diagnosis and treatment, but only as an aid toward better defining behaviors that might be influencing or building your tension headaches; your doctor may find it helpful if you show him or her your list.)

1. During the headache the muscles of your shoulders and the back of your neck feel tight.
2. Usually lying down and relaxing in a quiet room lessens the pain.
3. You are quick to lose your temper and seem to be angry at people most of the time.
4. There seem to be many frustrations in your life.
5. People think of you as "up tight."
6. During the headache your vision, hearing and balance are usually not affected, but you may feel dizzy.
7. The headache does not awaken you from a sound sleep.
8. Sometimes you get the headache after driving for long periods of time.
9. The headaches can occur at any time during the day.
10. Writing, typing or staying in one position for any extended time seems to bring on the headache.
11. The headaches seem to occur when you are under increased stress.
12. Sometimes massaging the back of your shoulders and neck seems to help.
13. The headache feels as though someone is tightening a band around your head.
14. Most of the time when you have a headache, you are too active to stop and relax.
15. Sometimes you feel depressed.

MIGRAINE

Most of you are familiar with the vascular headaches known as migraines. These headaches usually are broken into three classifications: classic migraine—occurring in about 10 percent of migraine patients; common migraine—seen in about 85 percent of patients; and cluster migraine—occurring in about 4 percent of patients. Many times a tension headache will occur before, during or following the migraine.

Classic Migraine

The classic migraine is usually preceded by a premonition of headache pain for approximately ten to twenty minutes and is usually followed by such manifestations as double vision, blurred vision and sometimes a distorted sense of balance or coordination. The pain is usually limited to one side of the head and is a pulsating, throbbing type of pain that may last from four to six hours. If the pain is not reduced, it may spread to other parts of the head and will change from a throbbing to a steady pain. Nausea and vomiting may follow in the later stages of a classic migraine.

Common Migraine

The common migraine is different from the classic migraine in that the preheadache stage is not associated with visual disturbances as in the classic migraine. The headache premonition may occur hours before the actual attack. Disturbances in thought, gastrointestinal disturbances and actual changes in the fluid balance of the body (such as excessive or retentive urination) may occur during the common migraine. The pain is steady, throbbing or aching and usually lasts longer than the classic type, from hours to days, affecting both sides of the head.

Cluster Migraine

The cluster migraine may be known by other names, such as migrainous neuralgia and histaminic cephalalgia. With this type of headache, there usually is no forewarning. The pain is predominantly on one side of the head and is commonly localized in the region of the upper cheek, eye and side of the face. It will usually recur on the same side of the face each time. The pain will become excruciating within a few minutes and may actually wake the individual after only a few hours of sleep.

The cluster migraine usually appears as a series of closely spaced attacks that can last upwards of eight to twelve weeks, with no attacks occurring for months to years. Each attack may last for only twenty to ninety minutes. Recent research has found that cluster migraines are more common in males.

STAGES OF THE MIGRAINE

The basic migraine attack can be divided into four distinct phases which display certain characteristics.

Stage 1: Preheadache:
The blood vessels get smaller in diameter (vasoconstriction). Some of these vessels supply blood to the brain and retina and, therefore, head pain may be preceded by certain visual disturbances or other symptoms such as speech difficulty, dizziness or weakness.

Stage 2: Headache:
This phase is typified by widening of the blood vessels (vasodilation). Arteries, veins, arterioles, venules and almost all branches of the external carotid artery are dilated, and as their walls stretch, the pulse increases, causing the throbbing sensation in the head to begin. The pain can become extremely severe.

Stage 3: Late Headache:
During the late headache stage, we find that the dilated blood vessels become very rigid and pipelike. The pain has now changed to a dull, steady ache and there may be localized tenderness of the scalp. Many people find that the pain in this stage is accompanied by nausea and vomiting, dryness of the mouth, sweating and chills.

Stage 4: Postheadache:
During the postheadache stage, pain is produced by muscular contraction generated by the anxiety and tension of the previous headache stages. The deep, aching pain of the muscular contraction part of the migraine headache may go on for hours or days.

MIGRAINE CONFUSION

Are you confused? There are many symptoms and an abundance of words to describe the migraine. I developed the migraine checklist to clear the air. If you find that a majority of the checklist items apply to you, then you may be a migraine sufferer.

MIGRAINE CHECKLIST

There are definite symptoms that go along with most migraines. Which fit your headache?

1. General tendency to withdraw from the immediate environment.
2. Mood changes.
3. Anorexia (lack of appetite).
4. Nausea and vomiting.
5. Constipation or diarrhea.
6. Photophobia (bothered by light) and sonophobia (bothered by sound).
7. Loss of color sense.
8. Localized or general edema (retention of water).
9. Diuresis (excessive urination).
10. Pulsing, throbbing pain, usually one side of the head.
11. Pain lasting for several hours.
12. Nasal congestion or rhinorrhea (runny nose).
13. Tearing.
14. Flushing of the face.

NOTE: As with any of the self-administered tests in this book, this is not meant to be a substitute for medical diagnosis and treatment. If you find that a majority of the symptoms from the migraine checklist fit your headache pattern, then let the checklist serve as an incentive to seek medical help and use the Pain Control Program to help relieve the discomfort.

Not a Disease

Headache, in itself, is not a disease. Headache is a symptom that may occur as a direct result of problems ranging from anxiety/tension to tumor. But don't let the word tumor bother you, since we find that the vast majority of headaches are symptoms of anxiety and psychological function.

After years of working with people who suffer from tension or vascular headaches, I have found that four basic personality make-ups seem to appear in chronic sufferers:

- Highly competitive
- Highly sensitive
- Perfectionist and meticulous
- Rigid in dealing with life situations

Realizing that one or all of these four factors may contribute to your headache is only the first step. Learning how to revise your behavior will go a long way toward reducing your headache discomfort. Here are some suggestions.

1. *Ventilate feelings.* Don't try to keep things inside. Talk about how you feel and let pent-up emotions escape. All of us need an escape valve.

2. *Don't let problems build up.* Find someone you can discuss them with. Using yourself as a sounding board isn't the most effective therapy. You need input and a chance to let other people know what's bothering to you.

3. *Reduce pressures.* Take a look at your life and work and isolate your pressure points. Then take positive action to let the steam out of them. Only you truly know where the pressures lie and only you can relieve them.

4. *Relieve emotional tension.* Survey your emotions and realize when you are most tense, and try to avoid the situations that set you up for emotional tension.

5. *Learn to relax.* The best way to accomplish this is to follow the Pain Control Program in this book. Since many of the causes of your headaches are learned behaviors, you can reeducate yourself to unlearn them.

6. *Headache diets.* Some foods or additives may be contributing to your headaches. Study Chapter Six, How Food Can Feed Your Pain, and start your elimination diet.

By combining environmental manipulation, ventilation of emotional conflicts and pressures, elimination of fatigue and learning a new way of coping with yourself and those around you, you *will* achieve positive results.

Your Headache Examination

Whenever you are bothered by headaches, you should consult your physician and obtain an accurate diagnosis. Determination of the type and cause of your headaches can be a crucial factor in choosing appropriate treatment for your particular problem.

The following guide will help you to understand better the headache examination and reasons certain tests might be given. Sometimes physicians do not take the time to inform a patient of the reasons for certain tests and this, in itself, may create anxiety and could possibly bring on a muscle contraction headache.

The first diagnostic step is gathering a complete medical history followed by a thorough physical and neurological examination. Specific attention is directed to the skull, cervical spine and shoulder areas. As the doctor examines your head and neck, he will inspect the area and perform palpitation, percussion and auscultation (listening). Sometimes the doctor may require a number of ancillary studies such as:

- Complete blood count
- Urinalysis
- X-ray of chest and skull
- Serology

Why Additional Studies?

Electroencephalography (EEG). May be used to detect certain diseases of the central nervous system.

Skull x-rays. X-rays of the cervical spine and skull are taken to rule out certain types of tumors or structural dysfunctions.

Brain scan. Used to detect lesions or tumors and may be used when the electroencephalography results are positive.

Spinal fluid examination (spinal tap). Used when there is a suspicion of intracranial infection or hemorrhage.

Angiography and pneumoencephalography. Used when there is evidence of some type of intracranial lesion.

Metabolic studies. Tests of urine and the blood are used to determine if there is any type of systemic (system-wide) cause for the recurring headaches.

Formal visual fields. This tests certain functions of the eyes and may be used to check for evidence of problems involving specific areas of the brain. This can also include sophisticated psychometric tests, such as the Halstead-Reitan.

CAT scan. A computerized analysis of the amount of x-ray absorbed by tissues that provides a detailed picture. Tumors, abscesses and bleeding are easily detected.

These procedures are by no means complete and each day new tests are being developed to help better diagnose and treat headaches. Hopefully they will give you an understanding of what to look for in an examination for headaches.

Some people have argued that they do not want to know why certain tests and procedures are being ordered by the physician and would rather remain in the dark. I totally disagree with this viewpoint since I think it is extremely important that you as the patient participate fully and actively in diagnosis and treatment of your problem. This is the only way you can take the responsibility for certain actions and behaviors that may be causing your headaches.

Success of any headache treatment is directly related to your understanding of the problem and your commitment to become actively involved in the treatment. The Pain Control Program will give you more answers.

Common Questions Your Physician May Ask You When Taking a History of Your Headaches

- When did the present headache or series of headaches begin?
- Can you remember the first headache you ever had?
- Do your headaches occur at night, during the day, in the morning, on awakening, or is there no particular time?
- Are you aware that you are about to have a headache attack?
- Are your headaches totally unpredictable?
- Before your headache, is there any nausea, vomiting or dizziness?

- Before your headache, do you experience light-headedness, disturbed sight or hearing?
- When you have a headache, is it on one side or on both sides of the head?
- How much time passes before your headache is at its worst?
- How long does it take for your headache to get better?
- Are you presently taking pain medication for your headache?
- What type of pain is it—steady, throbbing, knifelike, stabbing?
- Do your headaches seem to be triggered by loud noises or flickering lights, fatigue, alcohol or a particular food?
- Do you notice that headaches occur more frequently when you are upset or under extreme stress?

Additional Hints for Reducing the Headaches

1. Be Assertive with Your Headache. Realize that you need to become self-assertive; learning techniques such as saying NO when you want to say NO is extremely important. Specific techniques listed in the Pain Control Program will help you learn to become assertive, not only with your pain, but in all other aspects of your relationships.

2. Learn to Relax. Relaxation is absolutely the first step in overcoming most pain problems.

3. Stop Smoking. Ending your nicotine consumption is a vital and necessary step for anyone seriously seeking an end to his or her headaches.

4. Be Honest About Your Shortcomings. No one is perfect and learning to be honest with yourself will prevent a build-up of guilt that can lead to tension headaches.

5. Learn to Be Flexible. Don't be so unbending. You'll find that occasional flexibility will help reduce your headaches.

6. Don't Always Try to Be Perfect. No one is perfect all the time, so your chance of success, if this is your aim, is foreclosed before you start. Realize that you are human and will make mistakes, and be willing to learn from them.

Headache Summary

Vascular Headaches of the Migraine Type

Type of Headache	Onset	Duration	Type of Pain	Location	Frequency	Further Remarks
Migraine (Classic and Common)	Gradual	Several hours to several days.	Throbbing	Unilateral, temporal, in area covered by several cranial nerves	Periodic	Visual and sensory premonitory symptoms present in classic migraine; anorexia, nausea, vomiting
Cluster	Sudden	A few minutes to a few hours; average duration 30–90 minutes	Throbbing pain, intense and unbearable	Unilateral, in one eye or in the neck	Periodically recurring in rapid clusters	Flushing, sweating, rhinorrhea, lachrymation

Nonvascular Headache—Muscle Contraction (Tension) Headache

Type of Headache	Onset	Duration	Type of Pain	Location	Frequency	Further Remarks
Muscle Contraction (Tension)	Gradual	Variable—can be constant if not treated	Dull, constant sensation of pressure, tightness and constriction; varying in intensity	Bilateral, suboccipital (lower back of the head)	Episodic	Associated with sustained muscle contraction, usually as part of patient's reaction to stress

Headache Due to Sinus and Nasal Congestion

Type of Headache	Onset	Duration	Type of Pain	Location	Frequency	Further Remarks
Sinus Headache	Gradual	Length of inflammatory process	Deep, dull aching	Referred from infected sinuses to various facial areas: frontal— forehead ethmoidal— around eyes, bridge of nose sphenoidal— deep, behind eyes maxillary— cheek, upper teeth	Episodic	Pain intensified by stooping, coughing, or head-down position

7. Find Out If Your Diet Is Feeding Your Pain. Eliminate troublesome food.

8. If the headache in your temples is caused by high blood pressure in the arteries, it may be relieved by putting pressure on the sides of the bridge of your nose. Your finger restricts the flow of blood to the affected area and therefore decreases the discomfort. Runners who compete at high altitudes (over 10,000 feet) and climbers who attain very high altitudes often develop headaches because of the diminished oxygen in the air. Many of these people have found it helpful to wear a tight headband, which can reduce the pressure in the superficial arteries of the head and, therefore, reduce pain. In some Eastern cultures it is quite acceptable to walk around with a clothespin on the bridge of your nose to stop headaches.

9. Use the Pain Control Program to activate your built-in pain control system.

9

Back Pain

Yes . . . It Could Happen to You

No matter who you are—man or woman, adult or child, laborer or office worker—the chances are extremely great that you will suffer back pain at some time during your life. It may be only a temporary discomfort, or it could be the excruciating and incapacitating kind of pain that literally destroys your life.

According to medical estimates, some 80 percent of all people in the United States, Canada, Australia and Europe share this malady. And the cost is astronomic. Back problems account for more than 17 million physician visits each year in the United States and back injury has become our second most frequent health problem, second only to the headache.

Upright May Not Be the Best

Assuming the upright position separated us from most other creatures but it may not have been the best move for our backs. Weight is distributed evenly across the backs of animals that walk on all fours, but the same does not apply to us. By using bipedal motion (walking on our legs) we focus the brunt of our body weight on our low back area. Poor posture, lack of exercise, overweight and the ever increasing stress of daily life have placed additional pressures on this intricate organism we call the back.

Low back pain is one of mankind's most frequently experienced ailments.

There is no simple solution to back pain, although your physician should be consulted regarding any injury to your back. But there is something you can do. Improving your posture, performing your exercises and learning how to control pain through the Pain Control Program will be the keys to a healthy back.

Taking Your Back for Granted

We assume that back injuries happen only to construction workers, athletes and people who work for moving companies. This conception is totally wrong; back injuries can happen to anyone, at any time. It takes only a fraction of a second to injure the back and may take years to heal.

If you injure your arm or leg, that part of your body can be immobilized with a cast or splints and the healing process takes place quickly. This is not true with the back, for although we have back braces, it is almost impossible to immobilize the back totally without a body cast (a procedure not recommended for most back injuries).

Don's Repeating Injury

It was the beginning of summer and Don's lawn needed fertilizing. That night, after moving five sixty-pound bags from the store to his car and then spreading the mixture over his yard, he was in agony. Two days later he went to his doctor, who diagnosed the problem as a back strain and told him to rest for several days. He did and his back began to feel better, but Don was never given any exercises to help strengthen the muscles in his back and stomach, or any dos and don'ts to prevent further injury. When he rested his back felt great, but he was unaware of the damage he was causing by continuing certain daily activities that were interfering with the body's healing process.

If Don had been given the exercises in this book, along with the precautions to be used whenever a back injury has occurred, there is a very good chance that his prolonged suffering could have been eliminated. A good place for Don to start would have been learning how his back functions.

Anatomy of the Back

Starting with the basic anatomy of the back is essential to understanding the problem. The back is a wonder of anatomical engineering and is composed of a combination of hard and soft tissues. The twenty-four vertebrae of the spinal column, the five fused vertebrae of the sacrum and the four fused bones of the coccyx (tailbone) form the hard tissue. You have ninety-eight joints in the spine. Stress and strain on the vertebrae and joints will cause pain.

- CERVICAL SPINE. The top seven vertebrae make up your neck and support your head, allowing it to swivel, bend and rotate. Pain in these vertebrae may spread to the lower parts of the body.

- THORACIC SPINE. The next twelve vertebrae serve as attachment points for the twenty-four rib joints. Most ailments affecting this area are caused by poor health or improper posture.

- LUMBAR SPINE. Consists of five vertebrae that support most of your body weight. Poor posture, improper exercise or poor lifting habits frequently cause pain in this region.

- PELVIC SPINE. This is a wedge-shaped bone between your two pelvic bones and is held in place by strong ligaments. The last five vertebrae of the spinal column are fused together to form the triangular bone known as the sacrum. Poor lifting habits or improper exercise places a strain on your lower back region, causing your pelvic bones to rotate.

- COCCYGEAL SPINE. The small, segmented coccyx bone is connected to the bottom of the sacrum and serves as the attachment site for different pelvic muscles. Pain from this area may be a direct result of injuries or poor posture. Direct blows to this area may lead to serious injuries.

The soft tissues of the back are the muscles, ligaments and tendons that hold everything together and control movement.

Functions of the Spinal Column

The spinal column serves as the mainstay of the body's framework, as noted earlier. The spinal cord lies within its protective covering, with complicated networks of nerves reaching out to the farthest parts of the body. More functionally, the spinal column supports the head, provides attachments for the rib cage and anchors the pelvis. Ligaments (bands of fibrous tissue) support the column of bony vertebrae. Each vertebra is separated from the next by a fibrous disc that absorbs shocks to the spinal column.

Straight or Curved?

If you were to view the normal spine from the front, it would look straight, but viewed from the side, it has a series of four curves that enable it to carry weight and distribute stresses better than if it were absolutely straight.

Muscles and ligaments attach to the bony projections of the vertebrae and lend additional support and strength to the spinal column. Tendons are attached to the bone and connect to the muscles, which help to control all back movements.

The Curving Back

Most serious back problems are caused by injury and only about 10 percent are congenital (present at birth). Lumbar lordosis (swayback) and scoliosis, two of the most common acquired conditions, usually are not present at birth. Scoliosis is a lateral curvature of the spine that usually strikes teen-agers. It occurs with the same frequency throughout the world (twenty-five out of every one thousand young people), but is six times more prevalent in girls than in boys. Most researchers are at a loss to determine exactly what causes scoliosis.

Swayback appears to affect all age groups and is generally a result of excessive chest-out, stomach-in posture.

Getting Down to Basics

Diseases of the back are not as common as people would think. They include:

1. Tumors—malignant and nonmalignant.
2. Spondylitis—inflammation of the backbone.
3. Meningitis—infection of the spinal cord.
4. Arthritis—mostly osteoarthritis caused by age, inappropriate posture and prolonged stress.

All of these back maladies would be slighted if we were to ask a large group of people what they thought was the greatest cause of back pain.

Our society automatically thinks of the proverbial slipped disc whenever anyone mentions back problems. This is a misconception since only about 10 percent of back pain is caused by disc involvement.

The Mystery of the Discs

Discs are found between each of the vertebrae and are rounded, somewhat flexible pads containing a heavy gelatinous material surrounded by a fibrous cartilage. The discs act as cushions and shock absorbers and also prevent vertebrae from grinding against each other. There are basically two types of injuries to the disc.

1. Protruded disc. Due to extreme stress on the back, the disc has been pushed slightly out of place and may cause discomfort by pressing against a nerve in the area. In the past, many protruded discs were surgically treated, but recent advances in physical therapy have shown that an intensive regimen of exercise will help reverse the protrusion.

2. Extruded disc. The gelatinous nucleus of the disc herniates and breaks through its cartilage covering. Pain is caused by the piece of disc pressing against an adjacent nerve. Gradually the herniated disc loses its cushioning ability and the

disc space narrows. Extruded discs usually require orthopedic surgery to remove pieces of the damaged disc.

The Back's Number-One Nemesis

About 80 percent of all back pain may be caused by problems
with the muscles/ligaments and is a direct result of poor conditioning, general muscle weakness, decreased flexibility, poor
posture and poor lifting habits. Unresolved stress and the associated muscular tension may also be contributing factors to
back problems, and in our stressful society, they may be a major
factor in back pain.

Before you start the Pain Control Program, let's take a look
at some things you can do to keep your back healthy.

Keeping the Pain out of Your Back

"About one third of all workers in the United States perform
occasional, if not frequent, exertion that is hazardous—most because they are poorly matched to their jobs," explains Don B.
Chafin, Director of the University of Michigan's Occupational
Health and Safety Engineering Program.

Most people use their backs for at least 90 to 95 percent of
daily activities, but we are very lax in using this most important
part of our body in the proper manner. People who have good
posture give an impression of good health. Proper back habits
are largely a matter of practice and habit.

There are some commonsense rules for preventing back injury and reducing pain if you already have back problems. I have
listed dos and don'ts for many types of activities involving your
back and if you stay away from the don'ts and use the dos, you
will find your back remains healthier and, if injured, less painful. Take the time to copy these *back savers* into your notebook.

LIFTING

Dont's:
   Don't bend over with your legs straight.
   Don't twist while lifting.

Don't lift above the shoulder level.
Don't lift with the back.
Don't hold an object far from your body as you lift it.
Don't twist to set an object down.

Dos:

Do face the object you are lifting.
Do bend your knees.
Do lift with your legs.
Do hold the object close to your body as you lift it.
Do lift objects only chest high.
Do use the large muscles of your thighs when lifting.
Do pivot with your feet when turning an object to a new
   direction.
Do get help when the load is too heavy.
Do plan ahead to avoid shifts in the load.
Do make sure of your footing at all times.

STANDING AND WALKING

Dont's:

Don't stand in one position for too long.
Don't bend forward with your legs straight.
Don't walk with poor posture.
Don't wear high heels or platform shoes when walking or
   standing for any length of time.

Dos:

Do stand with one foot elevated on an object.
Do change positions often.
Do bend at the knees in order to keep the back straight.
Do walk with good posture, always keeping your head high,
   pelvis forward and toes straight ahead.
Do wear comfortable shoes that absorb the shock of walking.

SITTING

Don'ts:

Don't slump in your chair.
Don't sit in a chair too high to permit your feet to touch the
   ground.

Don't sit in a chair that is too far from your work.
Don't lean forward, arching your back, while you sit.

Dos:

Do sit in chairs that are low enough so that you can place both feet on the floor with your knees elevated slightly higher than your hips.

Do put something under your feet so that your knees are higher than your hips.

Do cross your legs or elevate your feet on a stool.

Do sit with your back firmly against the back of a chair.

Do use seat backs that are hard or firmly padded.

Do sit with your back firmly against the back of a chair.

Do use seat backs that contact your back four to six inches above the seat (not allowing the buttocks to slip under the back rest).

Do sit so that your lower back is flat.

SLEEPING

Don'ts:

Don't sleep or rest on a soft, sagging mattress or couch.
Don't sleep on anything that has a "hammock effect."

Dos:

Do use a firm mattress or lie on a firm couch.

Do sleep on your side with knees bent.

Do sleep with a pillow under your knees if you are sleeping on your back.

Do ask hotels or motels for bedboards.

Do use a bedboard under your bed at home if the mattress is not extra firm.

Do replace old, sagging mattresses.

DRIVING

Don'ts:

Don't sit too far from the wheel.

Don't have your seat back so far that you have to stretch to reach the pedals.

Don't drive for more than an hour without taking a five- to ten-minute break.

Dos:

Do move your car seat forward so that the wheel is easily reached and the pedals are accessible.

Do move your seat forward so that the knees are bent and slightly higher than the hips.

Do sit straight and drive with both hands on the wheel, thereby keeping your shoulders level.

Do stop every hour for five to ten minutes and get out of your car and perform stretching and flexing exercises.

Do check with your doctor regarding any orthopedic type of car seat that might be used for your specific back problem.

Do swing both of your legs out of the car when leaving and stand up as straight as possible.

Do try to avoid climbing and twisting into back seats.

MAINTAINING POSTURE

Remember

1. When standing, maintain the head in ideal position—head back, chin in.
2. When sitting, arrange your desk chair so that it will be easy to maintain the ideal head position.
3. Try to avoid the head back–chin up position or having the head forward in a flexed position.
4. Try to avoid tension within the neck and shoulder muscles by using your relaxation exercises or by occasionally rotating the head in a "no-no" movement with the chin close to the chest. Shrugging and relaxing the shoulders will also help loosen the neck muscles.
5. Make sure to sleep on a firm bed, using a soft or orthopedic type of pillow.
6. Regularly check the posture of your spine to make sure you are not in an incorrect position.
7. Regularly check your neck and shoulder muscles to make sure that they are not tense.

The dos and don'ts I have listed do not cover every possible situation in which you might find yourself. Therefore, common sense should be the best rule of thumb in avoiding further back or neck problems. Remember, always check with your doctor as soon as possible if back pain persists.

THERAPY THOUGHT: Good posture + commonsense body mechanics = Prevention of back injuries and less pain.

Activities to Avoid if You Have a Back Injury

Certain activities should be avoided, especially if they involve rough physical contact, twisting, sudden impact or direct stress on the neck or back. This list is by no means complete and I'm sure that you can add a few.

Tackle football	Touch football	Soccer
Volleyball	Handball	Racquetball
Gymnastics	Trampoline	Snowmobiling
Ice hockey	Weight lifting	Skiing

Specific calisthenics:

Twisting motions with the hips	Arching backward
Toe touching with legs straight	Leg raises
Sit-ups with legs straight	

NOTE: If you have a doubt whether you should be involved in an activity do two things:

1. Check with your doctor.
2. Use common sense.

In Summary

By knowing how your back functions and the origins of back pain, you will have a decided advantage over 99 percent of the people who experience back problems. KNOWLEDGE, PREVENTION, EXERCISE and the PAIN CONTROL PROGRAM are your best tools for insuring that your back will never put you "on your back."

As you proceed through the Pain Control Program, it is very important that you recall the dos and don'ts regarding your back. Take several pages of your pain notebook and write down some of the dos and don'ts that directly apply to your situation.

Even if you don't have back problems, DON'T IGNORE THIS CHAPTER. Understanding the basics of good preventative care of your back may save you from becoming a back pain statistic.

10

⊰§⊱

The Body's Built-In Painkiller

The young woman was lying on a table in the delivery room. Earlier, the pains of each contraction had shot through her body. But now, as the contractions increased in frequency and intensity, she began to feel less pain. She was totally aware of her doctor's every word and could see her husband standing next to her. She quickly followed each of the doctor's instructions and was able to answer his questions. As the pain increased and delivery drew near, she steadily became more relaxed and felt less discomfort. She was calm and at ease, totally immersed in the birth of her first child. She was using a form of self-hypnosis. Months before the birth of her child, she had undergone intensive training and had received posthypnotic suggestions regarding the pain at birth. As the pain increased, she automatically became more deeply relaxed and felt no pain, only a sensation of pressure. Even while under the posthypnotic suggestion, she was able to hear all her doctor's instructions and see her child immediately after birth.

Glen knew what was happening, but he was no longer inside his body. He was floating above himself, looking down and watching what was going on. He could see people changing the dressings on his horribly burned legs. Through the use of mental imagery, he was able to remove himself mentally from the scene and totally block the sensations of this extremely painful procedure.

Dirk felt the shooting pain in his left wrist after being tackled near the goal line. It was the fourth quarter and he didn't want to be taken out of the game, so he told no one of his injury. He had to run with the football again and the pain could be a handicap. By the time he ran back to the huddle, the pain grew less and less. By the time the quarterback was barking out the signals, Dirk's pain had totally disappeared.

Barbara was into the last mile of a 10,000-meter race (6.2 miles). Her lungs ached with each breath and she felt as though she couldn't go any farther. Something inside her pushed her toward the finish line. The pain in her aching leg muscles no longer registered in her mind. Her legs felt heavy, but the pain had disappeared several miles ago.

What Happened?

How were all of these people able to block their pain? None of them was given an anesthetic or painkilling drug. The answers had to come from within their own bodies.

The situations that I've just presented are by no means unusual. They all point to an elusive chemical within our own bodies which scientists have been searching for since the beginnings of recorded science. And yet, the first attempts toward stopping pain used chemicals produced outside the body.

Opium could be considered the grandfather of all painkillers and its use can be traced as far back as classical Greece. It is found in the unripened seed pod of the poppy. In 1803 Friedrich Serturner, a German pharmacist, created the first opium powder, which, from that time on, was known as morphine.

Until the nineteenth century, morphine's addictive properties and other negative side effects were largely ignored or unrecognized. When it became an established drug within clinical medicine, scientists began to study its positive and negative effects. Morphine was injected as early as the 1850s and already its severely addictive qualities were being documented. During World War I and World War II, morphine was used extensively to reduce the suffering of injured soldiers, leaving many of them severely addicted.

From the earliest uses of the poppy's seed pod to the multi-billion-dollar pharmaceutical business, opium has traveled a much scarred road. The well-known illegal drug heroin is another opium derivative, and because it enters the brain more rapidly than morphine, it can produce a higher state of euphoria, but the addictive side effects are devastating.

Many of you probably have taken codeine for pain, but most of you probably are not aware that codeine is a derivative of the opium poppy, although its potency is only about one-fourth that of morphine. However, they are both extremely addicting.

Whatever painkiller you may have taken or are presently taking, you should be aware that whenever artificial substances are introduced into the human body there is always the possibility of such reactions as addiction, the development of chemical imbalances and in some cases, damage to organs.

The Search for an Ideal Painkiller

For centuries man has searched the farthest corners of the world for the ideal painkiller. Dr. Everette May, formerly of the National Institutes of Health, has described an ideal painkiller as: "A drug that takes effect quickly, has long duration of action and, of course, one that has minimal side effects, such as respiratory depression, nausea, and drug dependence, and that can be as effective taken through the mouth as by injection." Unfortunately most scientists would be quick to admit that no such drug is presently known to man.

But the search for an "ideal painkiller" has not led to the development of a synthetic drug; instead, we are speeding toward probably the greatest discovery in pain relief—that each of us has a naturally produced analgesic (pain reliever) within our body.

Starting with the Placebo Effect

Basically, the placebo effect involves giving a patient a drug she or he thinks will help alleviate a symptom (particularly pain) when actually the treatment may be a sugar pill or sterilized water. This procedure is used to discover if the complaint can be resolved through psychological treatment rather than through drug therapy.

An example of the placebo effect can be found in an interesting experiment that has been duplicated numerous times, always with the same results. Patients who had just been through major surgery and were experiencing intense pain were divided into two groups. All the patients in the study were told that they would be given painkillers, but half were injected with sterile water. Approximately 35 to 55 percent of the patients injected with water, believing that they had been given a strong painkiller, reported a definite decrease in pain similar to that experienced by those injected with the actual drug. Those who believed they were being given pain medication, but actually were being given sterile water, had activated some internal mechanism that acted in the same manner as the narcotic medication. The "placebo effect" had activated the internal mechanism that mimicked the painkilling drug.

People who go through the Pain Control Program as inpatients at our hospital are given pain medication when they begin. This medication is equal to the medication they had been taking previously, but is in a liquid cherry-flavored base and is administered every four hours. The cherry-flavored base allows us to reduce the amount of medication without the patient's tasting any difference. At a certain point in the program, the patient is no longer receiving pain medication but is drinking only a cherry-flavored liquid. Many patients continue to report pain relief from the plain liquid. At this point we see the placebo effect taking place.

CASE

Norma M. was entering the second week of the Pain Control Program as an inpatient and during the morning session remarked that if it weren't for the pain cocktail, she didn't know how she would be able to go on. I gave her a quick smile and referred to the hospital chart on my desk. The chart showed that she had been on placebo for the past two days and, therefore, all the pain reduction she reported was being derived from cherry syrup. The placebo effect had initiated a painkilling mechanism within her body. I informed her of the placebo, and at first she was quite angry until I explained that she should be extremely proud of herself since she was now able to control the pain without medication.

The placebo effect may be our best proof that the body is capable of producing its own painkilling substance.

Endorphins: The "Morphine Within"

CASE

Randy S. banked the helicopter and started his low pass over the dense jungle foliage. He knew the clearing was just on the other side of the treetops and, once there, he could pick up the wounded and return to the station. His copilot, sitting to his right, joked as they skimmed the treetops at sixty miles an hour. The rain streamed off the windscreen, but he was glad, for the reduced visibility meant fewer snipers. Just as he cleared the final stand of trees, he felt the helicopter shudder and jerk, staggering under the impact of high-caliber bullets ripping into its unprotected belly. Randy shot a glance to the right just as his copilot was struck in the neck. The high-caliber bullet destroyed half the copilot's face and he died instantly. The control stick was heavy and sluggish in Randy's hand as he felt the searing pain shoot up his left leg. At the same time there was a sudden loss of breath and pounding in the side of his chest as if he had been kicked by a horse.

Randy knew he had been hit, but he was also aware of the fact that his was the only helicopter to pick up five critically wounded men in the clearing just below him. He saw the ground fire from his own troops forcing the snipers back into the woods. He made the decision to land and pick up the wounded men. As suddenly as the pain started, it stopped.

Randy picked up the soldiers and flew them back to the aid station. When he landed ten minutes later, the medics carried him from the helicopter and the pain suddenly returned in great waves of agony.

Randy was cited for his heroism and after recovering from his three bullet wounds returned to civilian life.

I find it extremely interesting that some mechanism within Randy's body blocked the pain response while he had to fly the helicopter, but as soon as he was safe on the ground, the mechanism stopped working and Randy felt the pain. Randy's built-in painkiller had saved not only his life but those of the men he had flown to safety.

Randy's example is not one in a million, for this same automatic painkilling response can be documented throughout history. Until now, no one knew why or how the response was activated.

A Worldwide Race

The discovery of the brain as the source of painkilling mechanisms came quite by accident. While studying drug addiction, Dr. Candace Pert and Dr. Solomon Snyder of Johns Hopkins University School of Medicine found that certain opium derivatives such as morphine and heroin would attach themselves to specific brain cell sites. The drugs fit into these sites (receptors) as a key fits into a specific lock. The question was immediately posed: "Were these opiate receptors present in man and animals for the use of some substances which would act as opiates and which were produced within the brain itself?"

The scientific race was on to discover what naturally produced substance would fit into the opiate receptors. Dr. John Hughes of the University of Aberdeen in Scotland isolated a chemical he named enkephalin, which was similar to morphine and could work as a key to the opiate receptors in the brain. When this chemical was injected into the brains of rats, it had a painkilling effect much like that of morphine or heroin. At the same time, as researchers the world over were obtaining similar results, a variation of enkephalin, named endorphin, was isolated. Endorphins were found to be released by the pituitary gland and have been estimated by some researchers to be 200 hundred times more powerful than morphine.

The latest development is the discovery of endorphins in the human placenta and amniotic fluid, giving rise to the theory that these built-in painkillers account for a woman's ability to withstand high degrees of pain during childbirth. The endorphins in the amniotic fluid may act as a natural sedative to the unborn fetus and allow the baby to withstand pain throughout the journey down the birth canal.

A Summary of the Research

Avram Goldstein, a pharmacologist and Director of the Addiction Research Foundation in Palo Alto, California, discovered that he could create an artificial (exogenous) key that could fit the opiate receptor lock located on the nerve cell wall. This artificial key, naloxone, could not open the lock. In other words, the key fit but was not able to act as a narcotic drug. You could call naloxone a "dummy key."

The use of naloxone has been an exciting development for emergency rooms since this false key is able to occupy an opiate receptor (lock) and therefore block true narcotics from the receptors (locks). Patients brought into hospitals in a near-death coma from heroin overdoses are given naloxone and the deadly effects of the heroin are quickly reversed. When using naloxone, an "in use" sign is essentially placed on each opiate receptor site and prevents the heroin from further affecting the body. Naloxone has also been found to be an effective indicator of narcotic receptor sites that can be used without having the subject endure the effects of the narcotic. When naloxone is tagged (mixed) with a safe radioactive material, a complete map of the opiate receptor sites can be plotted with x-rays.

Rats were used in an experiment to develop further proof of the endogenous (inborn) painkiller. The experiment was divided into two parts:

Part One. Electrodes were surgically placed in rats' brains. Their tails were painfully shocked. The rats showed a pain response and then their brains were given a mild electrical stimulation. The brain response was immediately stopped. The brain stimulation caused a built-in painkiller to be activated.

Part Two. The same rats were given an injection of naloxone before being painfully shocked. Unlike the first part of the experiment when the rats felt no pain after the brain was given electrical stimulation, they now felt the pain after electrical stimulation.

This experiment proved that the electrical stimulation of the brain had triggered the production of endorphins. When the rats were given the naloxone, the receptor sites were occupied and the built-in painkillers were useless.

Another most interesting experiment was conducted by the Medical College of Virginia in Richmond. Researchers there were attempting to determine if there was a link between acupuncture and the production of endorphins. They administered mild electric shocks to the teeth of thirty-five volunteers and measured how much electricity would cause the subject to indicate that pain was felt. Then, using an acupuncture point between the thumb and forefinger, each subject was given acupuncture for pain relief. The subjects were again shocked, but this time their pain threshold (the amount of electricity needed before they indicated pain) went up an average of 27 percent. Now the true test came; some of the subjects were given an injection of naloxone (endorphin blocker) and their pain threshold returned to the same level as before the acupuncture.

Obviously, the acupuncture had activated the production of the body's built-in painkiller. The injection of naloxone blocked the endorphins and, therefore, the acupuncture was ineffective.

From this experiment and numerous others, we now feel that the insertion of acupuncture needles into specific parts of the body may activate the release of endorphins into the central nervous system.

Dr. Bruce Pomerantz of the University of Toronto has conducted experiments showing that acupuncture diminishes the number of brain cells firing in reaction to pain. Following the removal of anesthetized animals' pituitary glands, he discovered that acupuncture provided no pain-relieving effect, although it had before the surgery. This led to the conclusion that the pituitary gland is a definite influence in the production of endorphins.

Production in the Pituitary

All activities of the human body are under the joint control of the central nervous system and the endocrine glands. The central nervous system is an immediate reactor, sending its nerve impulses, which may require immediate responses, to various parts of the body. The endocrine system works more slowly. Secretions from the endocrine glands are termed hormones and serve as exciters or messengers, carrying out their tasks in the far-reaching parts of the body. The pituitary gland, sometimes referred to as the master gland, secretes into the bloodstream substances that work directly with the central nervous system and may even activate other glands.

Endorphins are secreted by the pituitary gland simultaneously with the stress hormone ACTH. Once released, the endorphins seek out the opiate receptor sites to start the painkilling process. This interaction may provide an answer to why people under intense stress, in sports, military combat and emergencies, are able to withstand and sometimes not even notice pain. History records many such instances.

Where Is It?

The receptor sites located on the nerve cell walls can be considered the "locks," while the endorphin is the chemical "key." These receptors are highly concentrated in areas of the brain and spinal cord which have been traditionally associated with perception of pain. When endorphin is released directly into the bloodstream, it travels to all parts of the body and has easy access to the pain receptor sites. The internally produced endorphins fit into these locks and signal bodily reactions of relaxation, pain relief and a sense of euphoria. These locks may also be opened by opium-type keys such as morphine, heroin and other narcotics. The opium key not only fits into the opiate receptors, but may inadvertently open other locks, creating a generalized reaction within the brain cells and causing addiction.

The major advantage of endorphins is that they do not cause the generalized habit that opium derivatives do. The body's built-in painkiller (endorphin) is such a precise key that it fits only the opiate receptor lock and is nonaddicting.

An Answer from Acupuncture

For literally a thousand years, people have not been able to explain adequately the anesthetic or painkilling properties of acupuncture. We know that in many cases acupuncture has been effective in reducing or eliminating acute and chronic pain. I have found it curious that some people who receive acupuncture obtain immediate pain relief that may last from eight minutes to eight days, yet some people achieve permanent pain reduction from one acupuncture treatment. Acupuncture's painkilling properties may be explained by my associate, Dr. Dennis Harris, a physician and specialist in chronic pain who has trained in both the Chinese and European methods of acupuncture. Dr. Harris thinks that a needle inserted into specialized acupuncture sites may actually stimulate the neural pathways to signal the production of endorphins and, therefore, provide pain relief.

"For many years I've studied the relationship between mind and body in regard to chronic pain, and why such modalities as hypnosis and acupuncture appear to have painkilling properties. The discovery of endorphins as a built-in painkiller seems to answer the what, where and how. Of course, production of endorphin at the individual's internal command would be the ideal method of treatment delivery. No side effects, no expense or delay, just relief."

Synthetic Is Not the Answer

Drug companies and researchers have already been able to produce a synthetic form of endorphin, but have found it to be extremely addicting, a quality which naturally produced endorphin does not have.

Dr. Nathan S. Kline, a psychiatrist at the Rockland Research Institute in Orangeburg, New York, and Dr. Heinz Lehmann, a psychiatrist at McGill University in Montreal, have conducted studies of synthetic endorphin, but at the present time one injection costs $3,000. Obviously the price of the synthetic drug places it out of the range of most pain sufferers.

Hypnosis and Endorphin

Endorphins may be the key to the success of hypnosis in controlling pain. It is hypothesized that hypnosis directs the brain to produce the built-in painkiller. A person under hypnosis is in a very relaxed and highly suggestible state. During this period of relaxation, it appears that hypnotic suggestions for the reduction of pain automatically stimulate the production of endorphins. It is well known that people who are under stress are more susceptible to pain.

Another reason we fail to control pain when we are under stress may be that two chemicals (norepinephrine and ACTH), which are produced in large quantities at that time, suppress the action of endorphins.

Obviously, reducing stress and learning a good form of self-hypnosis can be an asset toward gaining pain control.

How Can I Use Endorphins?

The Pain Control Program is designed to teach you how to activate your body's production of endorphin to reduce your pain.

11

⋙⋙⋙

Alternative Methods
for Pain Control

No book on chronic pain would be complete without listing some of the alternative methods for controlling pain. The success of these procedures varies, and your physician may prescribe one or more. None of the methods listed in this chapter is used in the Pain Control Program, but some might be of benefit in particular instances.

The American health system has seen the rise in the phenomenon known as the second opinion. Before having surgery, many insurance companies are now paying for second opinions, to insure that the surgery is necessary and that a more conservative method of treatment might not be more appropriate.

The second opinion criterion should be applied to the alternative methods of pain control listed in this chapter. If you should have one of them recommended to you, don't hesitate to gain a second opinion. Although biofeedback and transcutaneous electrical nerve stimulation are not known to have side effects, some methods of surgery and injections for chronic pain are considered invasive (into the body) techniques and could bring about complications.

This chapter is strictly for your information and I can neither recommend nor criticize the techniques. It is my purpose solely to present them to you and let you and your doctor judge.

Surgery for Pain

Many of the patients I see in my practice have been subjected to numerous surgical procedures in an attempt to relieve pain. Unfortunately, surgery for the reduction of pain is not always successful and may, in fact, leave the patient with additional discomfort. Surgery, in most cases, is not a totally effective means for relieving an individual's pain.

Now or Later

Some patients endure excruciatingly painful surgical procedures in an attempt to burn a nerve, kill a nerve with alcohol or cut a nerve. All of these procedures are designed to relieve pain, but, in fact, many times the pain is eliminated only for a short period and, through some unexplained means, recurs at a later time. Once the sanctity of the human body is disturbed through surgery, all the apologies in the world will not take away the results of the surgical procedure.

A Frame of Reference

Surgeons are taught that surgery can be an effective answer to pain, when in reality very few surgical procedures actually reduce pain significantly. Although surgeons have shown a great deal of ingenuity in designing operations to relieve intractable pain, the statistics for success are very poor. I talked to one surgeon who had just finished a lumbar fusion for the relief of pain and his comment was, "The surgical procedure went perfectly, but who knows about the pain."

Surgery has been found to be a very effective means for alleviating pain derived from such acute problems as appendicitis, broken bones, tumors and infections. But the success of surgery for the reduction or removal of chronic pain is a completely different story and any surgery for the removal of intractable pain should be approached with extreme caution and a full knowledge of numerous failures.

Biofeedback

For thousands of years Oriental holy men claimed that they could consciously control their internal body functions. Western scientists consistently scoffed at these claims, but during the mid-1960s, biofeedback researchers proved that it is possible to control autonomic body responses on a conscious level.

Biofeedback is simply what the name implies, a method of learning to control body processes that ordinarily, without specific training, cannot be regulated voluntarily.

If you were told to drive a car at a certain speed without referring to a speedometer, the task would be very difficult; but with a speedometer you are able to gain feedback regarding the speed of your car and controlling it is quite easy.

Biofeedback machines have become extremely sophisticated and have fully entered the computer age. Universities are offering courses to train biofeedback therapists, and most health-related professions are realizing the true significance of biofeedback as a method for learning self-regulation.

Summary

While biofeedback may serve as an effective device for learning some methods of pain control, there are several prohibitive factors that need to be discussed. Biofeedback training should be undertaken only with direct supervision by a trained therapist. Therapy sessions are usually quite expensive and usually take place in the therapist's office. For most people, purchase of biofeedback equipment is not practical or advisable.

I have found biofeedback to be an effective tool when used as a starting point, but not as a therapeutic crutch. I prefer the built-in biofeedback of Pain Control Imagery; it is completely portable and can be practiced at any time, anywhere, and you are the therapist.

Nerve Stimulation

Transcutaneous nerve stimulation, or TNS, is the application of an electrical current through the skin to a peripheral nerve or nerves for the control of pain. This technique is relatively new to medicine, but has been widely accepted and positive results have been achieved.

Initially researchers felt that TNS units worked because they interfered with the nerve impulses carrying the pain messages.

This theory has been updated by the discovery of endorphins and at this point it is thought that TNS may be responsible for activating the body's production of endorphins through nerve stimulation similar to that effected by acupuncture. The units are quite expensive, ranging from $300 to $500 and must be ordered by a physician. Electrical current is generated within a small machine that can be worn on the belt and is passed along through wires to small rubberized electrodes. These electrodes are held in place on the skin by adhesive tape. Adjustments on the unit determine the amount of power and pulsations of current. This technique has several advantages; it is nonaddicting and does not have damaging side effects. The drawback is primarily its inconvenience. The machine is somewhat conspicuous and takes time to attach properly.

The use of this machine should be prescribed and supervised by a physician who is experienced in transcutaneous electrical nerve stimulation.

Acupuncture

We have already discussed this in relation to endorphins. The Chinese believe that acupuncture improves the balance between Yin and Yang and therefore changes the flow of life forces within the body. They describe the force of life as falling within twelve meridians (areas of the body). By inserting an extremely slender needle into specific meridian points, other areas of the body may be affected. Even with our tremendous fund of scientific research, no one is quite sure how or why acupuncture works.

Acupuncture's pain-relieving effect is usually short-term, but in some cases I have observed pain reduction that lasted as long as several months.

A Sharp Placebo?

Many scientists feel that acupuncture's cure rate of about 35 percent is similar to that of placebos. Of course, as you know, there is strong evidence to show that acupuncture actually stimulates the production of the body's built-in painkiller and thereby relieves pain.

If you decide to try acupuncture, be extremely selective in choosing the proper acupuncturist. It is my opinion that only an M.D. who has extensive training in this technique should be consulted. Unfortunately, there are many people who profess competency in acupuncture skills but have little or no technical training to reinforce their technique and knowledge. Your state medical association will be able to provide you with information regarding physicians who are certified in the use of medical acupuncture for pain relief.

The Treatment Merry-Go-Round

It is more the rule than the exception to find that a chronic pain patient may have been seen by up to fourteen different specialists. From TM to surgery, the person in pain seeks conventional to bizarre treatment in pursuit of relief. Unfortunately, most of the traditional treatments have been found to be generally ineffective for the long-term reduction of chronic pain and the constant shuffling from one specialist to the next may lead to the loss of time, money and confidence in the health-related professions.

To help you understand better how various specialties view chronic pain, I have developed a brief summary covering these areas of specialty.

ACUPUNCTURIST: A specialist who treats pain by the use of needles inserted in specified areas (meridians) of the body. Electrical current may be passed through needles, in which case the therapy is called electro-acupuncture.

ANESTHESIOLOGIST: This specialist usually deals with the patient during surgery. It is his or her responsibility to keep the patient insensitive to pain through inhalation of certain gases or by injection. He or she may also use injections to "kill" a nerve and stop the transmission of the pain signal.

BEHAVIORAL SCIENTIST: The behaviorist believes that pain is strongly influenced by social, environmental and emotional factors but can be modified through a plan of structured behavioral activities (changing the individual's interaction with people and environment).

BIOFEEDBACK THERAPIST: Pain may be resolved through the use of electronic monitoring devices to teach self-control of certain body responses, pain being one of them.

CHIROPRACTOR: The chiropractor bases his or her therapy on the conclusion that pain is caused by abnormal functioning of the nervous system and attempts to restore normal functioning through the use of manipulation, primarily of the spinal column.

NEUROLOGIST: Pain is a result of damaged or impaired neural pathways. Surgical or electrical techniques may be used in an attempt to interrupt the pain signals.

ORTHOPEDIC SURGEON: Most pain is a manifestation of muscular or skeletal system dysfunction and can be analyzed through x-ray procedures and treated by traction, immobilization or surgical techniques.

PHARMACOLOGIST: Most pain can be modified through the administration of pain-relieving drugs (analgesics).

PSYCHIATRIST: Pain may be a result of upbringing, life patterns and previous relationships.

PHYSIATRIST: Pain may be modified through electro-diagnostic techniques and treated by the use of physical therapy.

When in Doubt—Find Out

If one of the techniques in this chapter is recommended to you, by all means get a second opinion and go one step further. Visit your local library and read something about the procedure. Check with your local medical society. Don't allow any technique to be pushed upon you without your knowledge.

12

❧❦

Pain Imagery

To Each His Own

Each of us is capable of learning to reduce pain if given the proper training. For centuries Eastern societies particularly have persevered at pain control. The one common element in any philosophy of pain control seems to be the use of mental imagery techniques. In his book *Kamikaze*, Yasuo Kuwahara, a fifteen-year-old Japanese Kamikaze fighter pilot, detailed the techniques he used to cope with the pain inflicted during his grueling training as a Kamikaze. He used five techniques for blocking the pain: muscular relaxation, tension/relaxation, breathing exercises, massage and mental imagery. I found Kuwahara's use of mental imagery extremely interesting, especially what he called "the wonderful, blessed, great dark hole," where he could place all of the pain from his body. The fifteen-year-old fighter pilot actually was activating his body's built-in pain-killers to help survive suffering. While none of us is training for this type of career, suffering from chronic pain necessitates learning similar methods of control, but in a planned, easily understood, and tested program based upon scientific research.

The Foundations of Pain Control Imagery

The technique of Pain Control Imagery is based on recent scientific research.

Dr. C. Norman Shealy, internationally known neurosurgeon and founder of the Pain and Rehabilitation Center in La Crosse,

Wisconsin, has taught a form of pain imagery to over 1,200 patients who suffered from chronic pain. Dr. Shealy claims that pain imagery "is the number-one plan to stop pain." This leading pain specialist further states, "It's the single most effective therapeutic technique—bar none. It is more effective than acupuncture, drugs and other methods. And it works on headaches, backaches, arthritis and any other kind of pain."

This is quite a recommendation, and studies in our own Pain Center confirm Dr. Shealy's results; 83 percent of the patients who were taught Pain Control Imagery reduced their pain by 55 to 100 percent.

Dr. Irving Oyle, professor at the University of California Extension at Santa Cruz, further confirms Dr. Shealy's and my results through treatment on 1,000 patients of his own. Dr. Oyle, author of *The Healing Mind*, states, "It is the most effective pain reliever I know of. It really works on any kind of pain, from tension headaches to pain from muscles, joints and even from terminal cancer."

Dr. Dennis Jaffe, of the Department of Psychiatry at UCLA Medical School, reports that imagery becomes a way of communicating directly with your body. "You get pain relief by using only the power of your mind, your imagination." Guided imagery for pain control allows you to get in touch with the body's mechanisms for pain reduction.

In its early stages, pain imagery used relaxation as its main technique. Refinements in the method have been occurring consistently over the past ten years. Since the painkiller is coming from within the body itself, there are no detrimental side effects, an advantage over most medical procedures.

Relaxation, the First Step

Relaxation techniques are the basic building blocks of Pain Control Imagery.

Deep muscle relaxation is not only a refreshing experience but the first step in self-production of the body's own painkiller. You will learn that it is possible to control and relax even the smallest muscles in the body. When the body is in a relaxed state, mental imagery may be used to foster endorphin production. Without relaxation, Pain Control Imagery messages are blocked and never reach the brain's control mechanisms. Relaxation further places the body in a homeostatic state (everything working together harmoniously), which opens the body's channels of communication.

When we relax, certain changes occur within our bodies, although not all people will experience exactly the same responses. Here is a typical example of the changes that occurred in one patient:

1. Oxygen consumption was reduced; less energy was required to run the body.
2. The amount of carbon dioxide expelled decreased.
3. Respiration rate was reduced and thereby the body conserved energy.
4. Mucus flow in the digestive track increased (protecting stomach and intestine linings against acid irritation).
5. Blood flowed more freely through expanded vessels.
6. Pulse rate dropped 10 percent.
7. Blood pressure dropped 10 percent.
8. Skin temperature of hands and feet increased one or two degrees.
9. Blood flow to abdominal organs increased.
10. Metabolic rate decreased.
11. Brain wave activity slowed, but was more creative.
12. An overall sense of well-being ensued.
13. ABILITY TO PRODUCE ENDORPHINS increased.

Earlier in this book we learned that rapid, shallow breathing is associated with a state of stress and pain. Whenever you are relaxed, your breathing becomes slower and deeper and arises from the diaphragm.

Why Deep Breathing?

1. Deep breathing techniques can be used to supplement and complement other relaxation procedures you will be learning later in the Pain Control Program.
2. Deep breathing can be used to initiate a relaxation re-

sponse and may be a substitute for other methods of relaxation under certain circumstances. I find it helpful while standing in line at the checkout counter or while stuck in traffic.

3. Deep breathing will help you overcome fatigue. It increases your oxygen intake and allows carbon dioxide to be expelled along with other metabolic wastes.

A Form of Self-Hypnosis

Once you have learned the basics of relaxation through the Pain Control Program, you are ready for Pain Control Imagery techniques. These techniques are based upon a combination of two types of therapy: self-hypnosis and autogenic therapy. By bringing these techniques together, you are provided with what I consider the best and most proven method for internal body control.

Hypnosis

The first time I ever experienced hypnosis I was somewhat fearful. The therapist was a friend who was thoroughly trained in the use of hypnotherapy and spent time explaining exactly what was going to happen and what he was going to do. Even with these reassurances, I had the fear that he would have me do something foolish. But after my first hypnosis session, I couldn't wait to try it again. The feeling of total relaxation, calm and self-control was delightful and reassuring. There were no stars, nor a sudden blackout, only the soothing sound of his voice and a serene, cloudlike, floating sensation.

Following that initial session, I went into professional training to learn the technique myself. I have found hypnosis an excellent tool in helping others to learn pain control. Self-hypnosis is even better, since you become your own therapist. I recently used self-hypnosis to help me through the extraction of two wisdom teeth. The dentist used a minimal amount of Xylocaine to deaden some of the pain, and I proceeded to use self-hypnosis for time distortion and suggestions for controlling the bleeding. The time distortion worked extremely well. I told myself through self-hypnotic suggestion that the forty-five minutes I would spend in the dentist's chair would pass as if they were only five minutes. In fact, when I opened my eyes at the end of what I honestly thought was five minutes, the dentist informed me that both teeth had been extracted with only minimal bleeding. The posthypnotic suggestion to control bleeding had worked and the pain was controlled, so there was no need for even an aspirin later that day.

WHAT IS HYPNOSIS?

Very simply stated, the hypnotic state is a condition between being awake and being asleep. The main difference is that a hypnotized person can be active, walking, talking and even writing. In 1955 the British Medical Association, and subsequently the American Medical Association, developed what they considered to be a working definition of hypnosis: "A temporary condition of altered attention in the subject which may be induced by another person and in which a variety of phenomena may appear spontaneously or in response to verbal or other stimuli. These phenomena include alterations in consciousness and memory and increased susceptibility to suggestion. Further, phenomena such as anesthesia, paralysis, the rigidity of muscles, and vasomotor changes (sweating and blushing) can be produced and removed in the hypnotic state."

As you can see from this rather complex definition, hypnosis covers quite a wide range of self-controlled activities. While in the hypnotic state, your conscious mind is "asleep" and all suggestions are funneled to the subconscious mind. Hypnosis serves as a direct line of communication to certain parts of the brain, such as the pituitary, which produces endorphins.

For most people hypnosis is not something that can be learned in a matter of minutes; like riding a bicycle, it takes time and practice. During the Pain Control Program you will be given time and specific practice activities so that you can develop a good technique of self-hypnosis.

NOTE: The self-hypnosis process will be explained in further detail during the Pain Control Program.

Autogenics

Autogenic therapy was originally developed in Germany during the late 1920s by Wolfgang Luthe, M.D., and Johannes Schultz, M.D. This method has been widely used in Europe with excellent results and is presently receiving increased attention in the United States. When I was preparing my doctoral dissertation in 1974, autogenic therapy was part of my research. Imagine my surprise when, after searching through numerous libraries, I discovered that there were approximately 2,300 research papers regarding autogenic therapy—but only 10 in English! The situation has changed drastically since that time and autogenic therapy is taking its place within behavioral medicine as one of the most promising techniques for learning to control the body's response to pain.

In its basic form, autogenic therapy consists of six standard formulas used to suggest control of specific bodily functions.

These formulas are:

Formula 1—Heaviness
My arms and legs are heavy.
Formula 2—Warmth
My arms and legs are warm.
Formula 3—Calm heartbeat
My heartbeat is calm and regular.
Formula 4—Regular breathing
My breathing is calm and regular.
Formula 5—Abdominal warmth
My abdomen is warm.
Formula 6—Cool forehead
My forehead is cool.

When these are combined and the body responds positively, a homeostatic condition is created in which you can control certain body functions.

Combining the Three

After you have learned the basics of relaxation, self-hypnosis and autogenic training, you will combine them to form the foundation for Pain Control Imagery. Specific suggestions directing your body to produce endorphins will be taught to you during the practice sessions. And your own specialized pain formula will be developed.

Carefully follow all of the practice instructions and you will soon gain control over your pain. Here is the equation:

RELAXATION + SELF-HYPNOSIS + AUTOGENICS =
PAIN CONTROL → ENDORPHINS FOR PAIN
REDUCTION

Signal Without Suffering

When you become proficient in the use of Pain Control Imagery, you will be able to decide which pain stays and which pain needs to be decreased. "Why keep any pain?" you may ask. The answer is very simple. Pain is the body's warning signal, and whenever this alarm sounds, you should pay heed to it and make a decision as to whether you are going to use your Pain Control Imagery to reduce the pain, or check with your physician if it is a new and totally different type of pain. If the pain in your neck is the same one that has been there for two years and has been evaluated by doctors, then you may want to turn off the pain signal completely. But if the pain you experience is a new pain in your left knee, then Pain Control Imagery will help reduce the discomfort while you seek medical attention.

In summary, you can reduce the suffering, but keep the signal for your health.

Summing Up

1. Learning proper relaxation is the first step.
2. Self-hypnosis and autogenic training combine to form the core of Pain Control Imagery.
3. Anyone can learn Pain Control Imagery by following the proper training procedures.
4. There are *no* detrimental side effects to Pain Control Imagery.
5. By using Pain Control Imagery, you can stop the suffering, but keep the signal.

PART II

13

❧❦❧

Before You Start
the Pain Control Program

From the very primitive beginnings of man's attempt to al-leviate pain and suffering, people have been punished for not controlling their pain.

During the Dark Ages, the person who did not achieve any relief from his pain was thought to be possessed by evil spirits and rites of exorcism and bloodletting were used to extract or force evil demons from the body. The early 1900s saw the ad-vent of certain surgical procedures that were mostly performed under local or no anesthetic. Held firmly to the surgical table by large leather straps and menacing attendants, the patient faced an ultimate punishment for not getting better: death. Merci-fully, many of these patients died on the table, for those who did survive faced the almost inevitable infections and fever brought on by the lack of antiseptic postsurgical procedures. As medicine progressed, the patient's rate of survival increased, but patients were still faced with painful and risky surgery as a pun-ishment for not getting better.

Recently I was in an orthopedic surgeon's office while he was examining the back of a thirty-six-year-old postal worker. The man had been injured on the job six months earlier, and trac-tion plus bed rest had been unable to alleviate his ever increas-ing discomfort. The man pleaded with the doctor to help him gain some relief from the pain that was keeping him from his job and causing problems in the family.

Assuming his best professional tone, the surgeon informed

his patient, "If you don't get better and learn how to handle the pain, then I'll have no other choice but to operate." The bottom line: if you don't get better I'm going to punish you by operating.

The Pain Control Program has been designed to prevent you ever from being punished for not controlling your pain.

Before You Begin

You are about to embark upon the Pain Control Program, and if you were sitting in my office facing me, I would be explaining the Pain Control Program. "Beginning is easy—finishing is the true measure of commitment," I tell my patients in our first meeting.

Please remember, this is YOUR program, and by the nature of your pain and personality, you will customize it to fit your particular needs. All of the pain puzzle pieces will be set before you and together we will attempt to put them together, relieving the dilemma of pain! Therefore, the amount of pain relief you receive is in large part up to you, directly related to your commitment to the program. If you put in only an 80 percent commitment to pain control, then your result will be proportional. I will not be doing anything TO you, for I am only your tour guide on this trip, which, hopefully, will end in pain relief. No one is going to hold your hand; the responsibility is totally on your shoulders, but I will show you how to handle it successfully.

Before you read any further, let's make certain our lines of communication are open. Over the years I have developed specific objectives for this program that I want to share with you. Let's take a moment and review them. Copy the list into your notebook.

Objectives of the Pain Control Program

1. Reduction in the use of narcotic pain medication.
2. Desensitization to pain responses (relearning pain reactions).
3. Physical reconditioning.

4. Improved dietary habits.
5. Increased daily activity level.
6. Development of new behaviors to cope with pain.
7. Positive habit control.
8. Production of the body's natural painkillers.
9. PAIN CONTROL.

The Pain Control Program

I have designed the program to be effective over a two-week period. When the last day arrives, it will not signal the end of your program, but, rather, the transition into your Maintenance Program, which will continue indefinitely.

Each day of the program is designed with specific tasks and objectives. The program is purposely hard—just plain hard work and the newest and best methods for teaching your body to control its own pain. (If you should get discouraged with your progress, remember that this identical program would cost you from $2,500 to $8,000 in most pain centers within the United States, and could require up to six weeks in a hospital.)

Hard work and commitment are vital to successful pain control.

CASE

Jerry H. is a perfect example of 100 percent good intentions, but less than adequate commitment. Jerry was a chef who had been recommended to the Pain Control Program by his physician. Late one afternoon, Jerry was preparing for the evening meal when he stepped into a splash of grease. His legs flew out from under him and he fell backward, striking the small of his back against a low shelf. Jerry didn't think much of the injury until he tried to stand up and couldn't.

Three years and four back operations later, Jerry visited me. After examinations by our physician, psychologist and therapist, he was admitted to the Pain Control Program. Jerry was elated!

Everything went smoothly for the first three or four days, but then Jerry's personality began to change. As we applied more pressure, taking away many of his excuses and requiring more work on his part, Jerry balked.

"I want to do it, but I just can't. The pain hurts me too much. Can't someone give me something to get rid of the pain?" Jerry would say this repeatedly. The principles of the program were explained again and Jerry would progress nicely for a day and then slip back into his old, nonproductive patterns of behavior.

When Jerry was finally threatened with expulsion from the program, he decided to make a commitment and take the responsibility for learning the pain control methods. From that point on Jerry progressed each day, and by the end of the program, he was able to control approximately 30 percent of his pain. One month after the program ended, Jerry was able to control over 60 percent of his pain, and the last I heard from him he was doing even better and was back at work.

THINK ABOUT JERRY WHEN YOU FEEL YOURSELF LOSING COMMITMENT.

Giving a Helping Hand

People who are important to us and with us much of the time are called significant others. They play a direct role in how you learn to cope with pain.

Here are some simple rules that should be followed by your significant others. The best method is to write down these rules and give copies to each significant other in your life. Let them know that you consider their following these rules to be very important in your battle against chronic pain.

Rules for Significant Others

DON'TS

- Don't constantly ask how the other person feels.
- Don't make comparisons with other people.
- Don't do everything for him or her.
- Don't inadvertently create a cripple.

- Don't become a "professional" nurse.
- Don't make excuses for him or her.
- Don't use his or her pain behavior as an excuse for your behavior.

DOS

- Do let the person with a pain problem know that you care about and love him or her.
- Do reinforce and compliment him or her for behaviors unrelated to pain.
- Do be understanding of the difficulties involved in reducing narcotic pain medication.
- Do help him or her with the Pain Imagery exercises.
- Do help him or her with the physical reconditioning exercises.

When you give this list to one of your significant others, don't forget to add any dos or don'ts that apply to your particular situation. Try to be as forceful as you can when you tell people to follow the dos and don'ts. If you are wishy-washy, they'll follow the rules in a wishy-washy manner.

Who Fails?

Unsuccessful completion of the Pain Control Program is not a topic I like to discuss. But unfortunately, some people, mostly because of their attitude, set themselves up for failure even before they begin.

If you can find yourself in any of the three following descriptions, don't despair, it's not too late, but you must make some changes in your behavior before you start the program.

TOM TOMORROW

"I'll begin my program tomorrow!" Sound familiar? Well, if it does, you may be one of the "Tom Tomorrows" who insist their programs of exercise, weight loss or other forms of self-improvement will definitely start tomorrow. Unfortunately, tomorrow is put off until the day after and then their tomorrows never evolve into todays. Don't be a "Tom Tomorrow." Decide upon the day you are going to start your program and stick to it.

JANICE JOINER

Janice has headaches and she's already tried eight different programs for pain relief, covering everything from biofeedback to acupuncture. After several visits to such programs, Janice becomes disillusioned by the absence of "miracle cures" and drops out to join the next program. She's quick to sign up, but almost never follows through. Her road to pain relief is paved with good intentions, but no results. The Janice Joiners usually are quite well read and have an abundance of factual information regarding various techniques, although their lack of follow-through prevents them from learning or using the techniques. Carefully reading the Complete Pain Encyclopedia is only the starting point of the race against pain. The Pain Control Program and Maintenance Program will be the true measure of your success.

RANDY AND RUTH RATIONALIZATION

"Why should I stop taking pain medication that my doctor prescribed?"

"I know some people who take lots of pain medication and they're still all right!"

"I would start the Pain Control Program, but I don't know if I have the time."

"I probably couldn't learn self-hypnosis anyway." The rationalizations and self-justifications go on ad infinitum. Making excuses for not taking the responsibility for learning pain control can be very easy. When you begin to believe these excuses, rationalization becomes a pattern of behavior. If you've come this far in the book, then there's no excuse or rationalization that could justify not completing the Pain Control Program.

There may be a little of Tom, Janice, Randy and Ruth in all of us. That's okay, just as long as it does not interfere with your learning to control the pain.

Every Day

The Pain Control Program is designed to be used on a daily basis. Proper planning of your time will insure greater success than will a great deal of enthusiasm with poor planning. Each day's program is broken into two parts—the morning and evening sections. During the course of your daily activities, you will be asked to practice certain aspects of your Pain Control Imagery each hour, but the bulk of your time will be devoted to the morning session and the evening session. Don't leave everything until late in the evening, for this just makes you hurry, perform some of the exercises poorly and lose some of the pain control benefits.

You will need to copy the Daily Report Form onto fourteen pages of your notebook and keep track of your daily progress. This serves as a positive reinforcer and helps you overcome negative behaviors that have been prolonging your pain. Proper record keeping helps to prevent you jumping ahead, falling behind or skipping one of the day's activities and finding out that you've forgotten one of the exercises as you are turning off the bedroom light at the end of the Johnny Carson show. (Since you are the only one who truly knows your schedule, you will have to take the responsibility for planning each day.) Most people find it helpful to read over the next day's activities the night before. This allows for proper scheduling of your time.

Dos and Don'ts

DON'T:

Skip a day.
Put off your complete program until late in the evening.
Give up if your results aren't immediate.
Try to short-cut the program.

DO:

Plan for a specific time each day to work on the program.
Read the next day's lesson the night before.

Record the Pain Control Imagery the night before.
Keep your diary up to date.
Think positively about your ability to control pain.
Use the Maintenance Program.

The Maintenance Program

After you complete the fourteen-day program, it is important for you to maintain your pain-reducing skills and further increase your ability at pain control. Your use of the Maintenance Program should last indefinitely. As with the Pain Control Program, set a specific time each day for your programmed activities, being careful not to skip a day just because the pain has been reduced. Your faithful adherence to this program is necessary for a continued ability to activate the body's built-in painkiller.

Not for a Lack of Ability

Those of us who have suffered chronic pain often lack confidence. "I won't be able to do it," "It's not possible," are statements heard over and over. Because of past misconceptions leading you to believe that you cannot control certain aspects of your body's functioning, the Pain Control Program will require you to change any previous negative thinking. If you enter the Pain Control Program with the dark cloud of failure hanging over your actions, you may set yourself up for still another failure.

The word "can't" has to be eliminated from your vocabulary before you begin the Pain Control Program.

Quick Tips

Probably the most important lesson of the Pain Control Program is that you must believe in yourself and the built-in ability you have to control discomfort. When in doubt, reread the following suggestions, review them from time to time and keep moving forward.

- Always proceed in small, easily achievable steps. Your start in the Pain Control Program is planned to be slow and solid with the main purpose of long range success.
- Don't forget to give yourself rewards. Pat yourself on the back when you have a success and take the credit, for you did it all by yourself!
- Remember, no program works all the time and if you should have a slight setback, don't become discouraged. Analyze your situation and seek out any flaws in your planning. I don't expect you to get everything right the first time!
- Don't be ashamed to ask for help when you need it. My address is listed in the back of this book and all letters will be answered. There may be a simple answer to your question that will allow you to gain a greater degree of success in your program, but you must ask in order to receive an answer.
- Don't hesitate to seek out a qualified physician if you should notice a completely new pain or physical symptoms that have not been diagnosed. If you don't have a family physician, seek advice from your state medical association. They will be glad to refer you to the proper specialist.
- Because I have had to use the "shotgun" approach in this book, some of the examples may not have applied to you. Please don't think they were wasted, for awareness of problems that could affect you in the future and stopping them before they get started can be good preventive medicine. Remember, the choice or change is strictly your decision.
- Always keep in mind that reeducating your body to produce its built-in painkillers at your command will take time and repeated practice. Be patient with yourself and give Pain Control Imagery a chance.

It's Contagious

Through experience with my patients and myself, I've found that once you gain control over one part of your body, which you thought impossible, the effect becomes contagious and soon you learn that other body functions can be controlled as easily.

The ability to control body functions can be turned into a contagious blessing. If someone can be taught to increase or decrease heart rate, decrease blood pressure, increase skin temperature, dilate or constrict blood vessels, then reducing the amount of pain experienced is a very reasonable request of the body.

MAKE THE PAIN CONTROL PROGRAM ONLY THE BEGINNING!

14

⊷§§∾

Exercising Away Pain

Why Exercise for Pain Control?

Physical exercise is probably the most important aspect of your Pain Control Program, other than the Pain Control Imagery.

NOTE: Be sure to check with your doctor before you start the exercise program. Show her or him the exercises and make sure that none of them interferes with any of your physical problems. The exercises have been designed to be compatible with most people's abilities.

Exercise Checklist

Read through each one of the statements and write down in your notebook any that apply to you.

1. I do not have any regular exercise program.
2. I should lose weight.
3. Climbing a flight of stairs causes me to breathe faster.
4. I seem to tire easily.
5. I don't like the way I look physically.
6. Whenever I'm active, the next day I'm so sore I can barely move.
7. I don't feel physically strong.
8. I avoid physical activities.
9. Sometimes I'm too tired for sex.
10. People stare at me.

Even if you identified only one statement, you are in need of an exercise program. The exercise program found in this book has been designed to help you gain a level of physical and emotional fitness that can last a lifetime.

Spring Training for Pain Control

Each year during spring training for baseball, football and other sports, athletes experience the muscular pain of conditioning; as conditioning develops, pain decreases. Unless we are physically active each day, our muscles are in a state of semi-contraction and stretching them out will cause a certain amount of discomfort. When you are involved in physical activity or are in chronic tension, stress or pain, your muscles are in contraction. This limits the amount of blood that can flow into that muscle and bring with it a relaxing supply of oxygen. The tensed muscle also releases minute amounts of kinins, warning messengers that act directly on special nerves that carry signals of pain. When the muscle is in a prolonged state of contraction, kinins signal the body to initiate a relaxation phase, allowing an increased flow of blood and introducing new oxygen that carries away these pain-signaling by-products (kinins) of the muscle contraction. You can easily understand how a person who suffers from tension caused by chronic pain may actually be increasing discomfort by not exercising.

Why Stretching?

As part of the exercise program, you will be performing stretching activities along with muscle strengthening. Stretching has the beneficial effect of increased blood circulation and muscle metabolism. Stretching also relaxes the muscles, tendons and joints. Following your stretching exercises, you will notice the warmth of increased blood flow.

Lack of Activity

"If I move, I hurt; therefore, the more I move, the more I'll hurt." This statement is commonly made by people suffering from pain. They are under the misconception that activity will bring about increases in pain, so they stop any kind of movement at all and actually initiate more pain through lack of activity. This avoidance becomes a major goal in their lifestyle.

If you were to sprain your wrist, then you could expect an increase in pain when you tried to use the wrist right after the injury; this discomfort prevents you from further traumatizing or damaging the area. The warning signal of pain has helped you prevent injury. This is not always true with chronic pain and you must consciously retrain yourself to become active again.

CASE

Sandy B. has suffered for years from unrelenting back pain. When she first began the exercise segment of the Pain Control Program, there was an increase in discomfort in the area of her back and other muscles, too. She immediately stopped her exercising after the first day and came to me with tears in her eyes. I explained to her that the increase in discomfort was a normal process, but I saw from the look she gave me that my explanation was not totally believed. I had her talk with other patients who had gone through the program and they also related stories of increased discomfort and soreness at the start of their programs and informed her that this discomfort decreased after the first week as their bodies accommodated to the exercise program.

With only half a heart, Sandy started her exercise program for a second time. She was not convinced of what she had heard until the eighth day, when she came into my office with an ear-to-ear smile. "The program's really working! I don't feel sore anymore. I'm going to do my exercises from now on!" Sandy was hooked, but if she had given up on first impulse, her chances of learning how to control pain would have been extremely slim.

Your Program

Now that you know the why, here's the how. The exercise program that you'll be participating in during the Pain Control

Program is designed for your benefit. The specific objectives of this program are:

· Increased muscular strength.
· Increased muscular endurance.
· Increased flexibility.
· Increased blood flow to the muscles.
· Increased elimination of waste materials from the muscles.
· Increased ability to deal with stress.
· Increased positive self-image.
· Increased capacity for stretching.

· Decreased production of kinins.
· Decreased muscular fatigue.
· Decreased muscular tightness.
· Decreased risk factors in heart disease.
· Decreased joint stiffness.
· Decreased inactivity.
· Decreased pain.

It should be easy for you to see the basic relationship between the Pain Control Program's exercise phase and learning to cope with your pain. One of the best places to start is your stomach.

Why Strengthen Your Stomach Muscles?

You'll notice that many of our exercises are designed to strengthen the abdominal or stomach muscles. The reason is twofold: by making these muscles stronger, you can help prevent low back injuries and relieve some of the low back pain you may presently be suffering.

The abdominal muscles are the only group of muscles that can take over some of the load placed on the lower back. They consist of large bands of muscle fiber that stretch completely around the stomach and connect in the middle of your back. When the abdominal muscles are weak, there is a high risk that any extra load placed on the lower back will not be helped by the abdominal muscles and, therefore, will lead to back injury.

NOTE: The abdominal exercises will also help you to "flatten your tummy" and that never hurts any of us.

STOMACH-STRENGTHENING EXERCISES

HELP	HELP	HELP
prevent	reduce	you to
reinjury	pain	look better

DONT FRET: IT'S NOT TOO LATE

Strengthening abdominal muscles is a small but extremely important aspect of the exercise format within the Pain Control Program. You are going to be strengthening and stretching muscles of the back, stomach, arms, legs and neck. Developing good strength, stretching and flexibility is not gained overnight; it is a process that takes time and perseverance.

Getting Started

As with any exercise program, there are certain ground rules and precautions that must be observed. You should have had a recent physical by a physician, and, as cautioned earlier, shown the doctor these exercises. Once you have his or her okay, you are ready to roll.

Knowing the ground rules is the first step. Each one of these rules has been carefully thought out, tried and proven. Follow them faithfully.

Ground Rules for Exercising

1. Exercise every day. A hit-and-miss program has no benefit.
2. Set up a specific time, as noted. Exercise twice a day, preferably once in the morning and once in the evening. Each of us has optimal physical activity periods during the day; usually the morning and afternoon are the best.
3. Perform your exercises on a firm yet comfortable surface and do them in the same place each day.

4. Wear comfortable, loose clothing when exercising.
5. Always begin with a brief relaxation exercise. Perform the exercises slowly and smoothly. Don't rush or use jerky movements.
6. Remember that the mild stiffness or soreness you feel after you first exercise will begin to disappear in three or four days.
7. Don't forget to record your progress.

THERAPY THOUGHT: *If any of the exercises give you significant discomfort that does not disappear after several days, discontinue that exercise and check with your physician.*

What the Patients Say

Here are some statements of pain patients regarding the exercise program.

- "I feel more alert and less depressed since getting involved in exercising."
- "There's a spring to my step. I don't hobble along anymore."
- "I feel good about doing something about my body."
- "Since I began exercising, I've lost weight and now can look in the mirror without feeling ashamed."
- "I feel energized and my pain isn't so important anymore."

After going through the Pain Control Program, you will be able to add your own statements.

The Daily Exercises

NOTE: Although the illustrations of the exercises depict female figures, all exercises are equally appropriate for men.

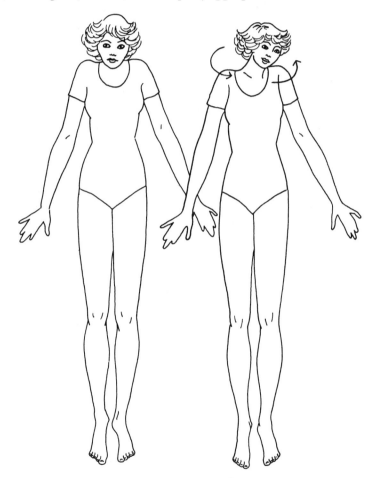

1. HEAD ROLLS. Sit or stand erect and let your chin drop to your chest. Gently roll your head in a full circle, first completely around to the right, then to the left.

Results: This exercise is good for neck, shoulder and headache pain.

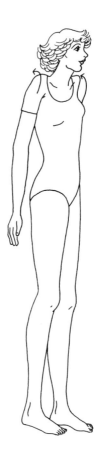

2. SHOULDERS UP AND DOWN. Stand up straight, with feet slightly separated, arms hanging loose at your sides. Shrug your shoulders in a circle by bringing them up as high as possible, then as far back as possible, pulling the shoulder blades strongly together in the back, then relaxing the shoulders. Many people tend to thrust the head forward while doing this exercise, and this should be avoided. Hold your head up, and your neck as straight as you can.

Results: This exercise will loosen muscles of the shoulders and neck.

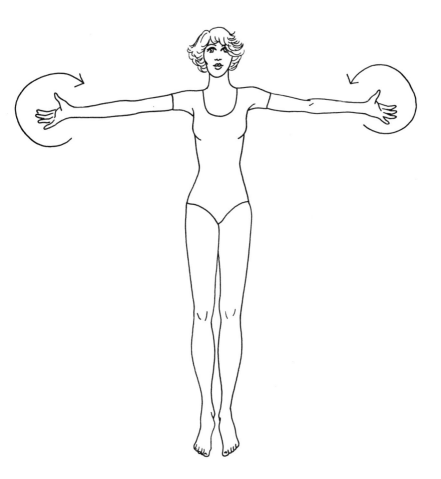

3. ARM CIRCLES. Stand erect with arms extended out at shoulder height with your palms up. Describe small circles backward with the hands while keeping head erect. Reverse, turn palms down and do small circles forward. As you become more proficient at this exercise, increase the size of the circles.

Results: This exercise is good for reducing pain in the shoulders, shoulder blades and upper back.

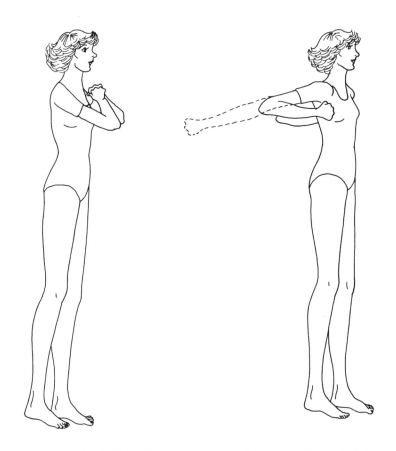

4. BACK STRETCHER. Stand with your feet slightly apart, arms raised to shoulder height, elbows bent and hands in front of your chest. Keeping your elbows bent, bring your upper arms back and tighten your shoulder blades. Straighten your elbows and swing both arms straight back, keeping them at shoulder height and bringing the shoulder blades together. When you bring your whole arm back your thumbs will be pointing toward the ceiling. Check to make sure that your head does not jut forward while doing this exercise.

Results: This exercise stretches the chest muscles and reduces postural pain.

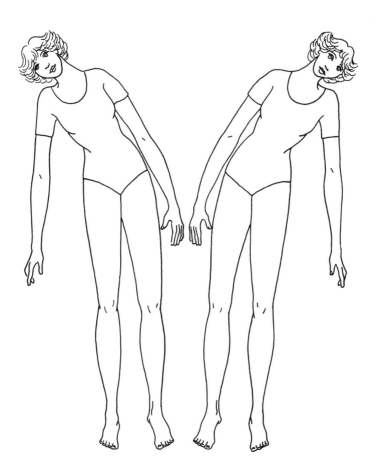

5. BACK BENDER. Stand with your feet between 1½ and 2 feet apart, hands hanging at sides. Bend to the right, sliding the right hand down along the outside of the right leg as far as possible. Straighten up. Repeat, bending to the left. Many people will bend forward slightly while doing this exercise. This is wrong. Try to keep the body in a straight line from front to back while bending to each side.

Results: This exercise stretches and strengthens the muscles and joints along the side of the spine and reduces back pain.

The Abdominal Five

All of these exercises are excellent for strengthening the abdominal muscles and reducing low back pain.

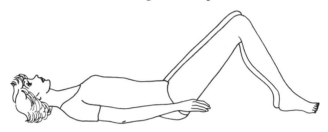

6. PELVIC TILT. Lie on back with knees bent and feet flat on the floor. Tighten abdominal muscles, pinch buttocks together and press low back flat against floor. Hold five seconds. Relax.

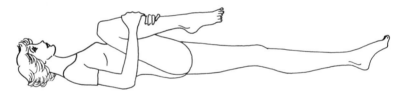

7. SINGLE KNEE TO CHEST. Lie on back with knees bent and feet flat. Grasp one knee with hands and pull toward chest. Hold five seconds. Relax. Repeat with the other knee.

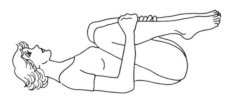

8. DOUBLE KNEE TO CHEST. Lie on back with knees bent and feet flat on floor. Grasp both knees and pull toward chest. Hold five seconds. Relax. Repeat.

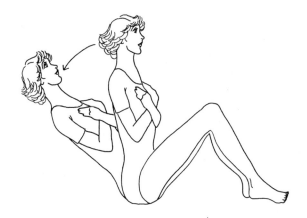

9. CURL DOWNS. Sit with both knees bent, feet flat on floor and arms folded across chest. Feet must be stabilized by hooking them under a chair or bureau. Lean back slowly toward the floor until you reach an angle of 60° with the floor. Hold for five seconds. Relax. Repeat.

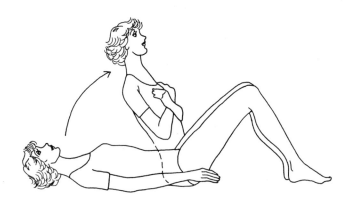

10. CURL UPS. Lie on back with knees bent, feet flat on the floor, arms folded across chest. Raise head and shoulders to a ⅓ sitting position. Hold for five seconds. Relax. Repeat.

Optional Walking/Running

Over 13 million people have taken to the new American craze of walking or running. The advantages of such activity are numerous: improved oxygen consumption during exertion, lowered heart rate while resting, improved relief of accumulated psychological stress, increased muscle tone, reduced blood pressure, release of muscular tension (reducing pain) and increased heart and lung efficiency.

Before you begin any walking or running program, always check with your doctor. Walking/running is not a mandatory part of your Pain Control Program, but may be added as an optional activity. If you desire, riding an exercycle may be substituted for walking/running (see Appendix Two).

WALKING/RUNNING TIPS:

1. Try to walk/run in an upright position with your head up. Don't watch your feet.
2. Keep your arms, shoulders and neck muscles relaxed.
3. Land on the heel of your foot and rock forward to drive off the ball of your foot.
4. Use a comfortable stride.
5. You may want to walk or run on soft grass to reduce the pounding shock to your body.

STARTING THE PROGRAM

1. Begin with short walks to build your endurance. Gradually increase the time and distance.
2. Whether you run or walk, don't focus on speed. Take your time and move at a comfortable pace.
3. Practice relaxing while you run or walk. Continuously check for a build-up of tension in your muscles, especially the neck and shoulder muscles.
4. Try the "talk test" to find the right speed. If you are too out of breath to talk, you are going too fast. Slow your pace.

NOTE: If you develop pain or other uncomfortable symptoms, slow down or stop. If they continue, see your doctor immediately.

For further information regarding walking or running programs, contact your library or a local jogging club.

Exercise Summary

All of these exercises are to be performed twice a day except for the walk/run, which is optional (once a day). The proper number of repetitions for each exercise is shown on each day of the Pain Control Program.

1. Head Rolls
2. Shoulders Up and Down
3. Arm Circles
4. Back Stretcher
5. Back Bender
6. Pelvic Tilt
7. Single Knee to Chest
8. Double Knee to Chest
9. Curl Downs
10. Curl Ups
11. Optional Walk/Run

15

◆§§◆

Getting Started

Last stop before the Pain Control Program! Here is the final countdown of instructions and self-evaluations.

- The Personal Pain Diagram
- Pain Influence Profile
- Daily Record
- Drug Record
- How to Make Pain Control Tapes
- How to Start Each Pain Control Imagery Session

Diagraming Your Pain

Over my years of working with chronic pain patients, I've learned one of their most difficult tasks is to describe their pain. That's why I developed the Personal Pain Diagram. Trace or copy the diagram into your notebook and fill it in, using the key provided. At the end of seven and fourteen days you will be filling out identical diagrams and checking for changes in your pain patterns.

PAIN KEY:

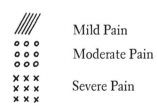

/////	Mild Pain
o o o o o o o o o	Moderate Pain
x x x x x x x x x	Severe Pain

Personal Pain Diagram

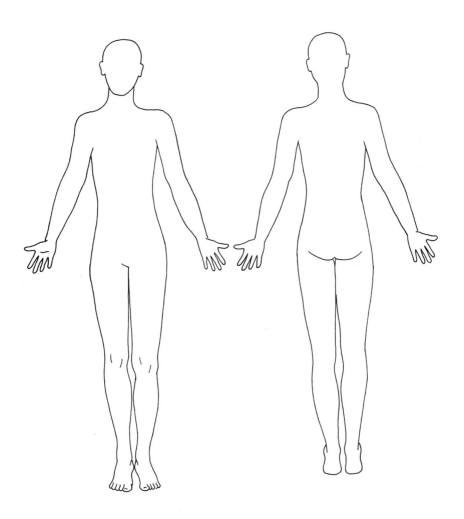

Pain Influence Profile

Some activities are difficult for a person with a pain problem. It will be helpful for you to indicate how each of the following activities affects your pain, and to what degree. You will fill in the Pain Influence Profile three times—on Day One, Day Fourteen and at the end of your first month on the program—so it will also give you a record of your progress. Place the appropriate value in the box next to the item. NA (Not Applicable) = 0, Mildly = 1, Moderately = 2, Severely = 3, Cannot do because of pain = 4.

Copy the form into your pain control notebook. We will use the profile more than once.

	Day One	Day Fourteen	One Month
1. Dressing—putting on shoes and hose.			
2. Grooming—wash, dry hair, shave, shower, bathe.			
3. Hanging up or putting away clothes.			
4. Meal preparation.			
5. Cleaning, vacuuming, dusting, making beds.			
6. Sexual activity.			
7. Picking up objects from floor.			
8. Sports, recreational activities (tennis, golf, bowling, etc.).			
9. Laundry—handwashing, washer/dryer, wringing, ironing.			
10. Grocery shopping.			

	Day One	Day Fourteen	One Month
11. Reaching shelves—above or below counter.			
12. Mopping or sweeping floors.			
13. Driving.			
14. Dancing.			
15. Washing/drying dishes.			
16. Minor home repairs, use of small tools.			
17. Care for garden, mowing lawn.			
18. Lifting.			
19. Bending.			
20. Walking.			
21. Sitting.			
22. Use of stairs, steps.			
23. Typing.			
24. Watching a movie.			
25. Reading.			
26. Writing.			
27. Jogging.			
28. (add your own).			
29.			
30.			
Total			

What Does the Score Mean?

After you have completed the profile, add up your score. The total is your Activity Index. Take the profile again after the fourteenth day and after one month. You will be pleased to see your score go down. Pay careful attention to activities in which your pain is decreasing and try lowering it further. Scores that do not change indicate areas for increased attention.

Your Pain Rating

Each day you are to rate your general level of pain after the morning session and after the evening session. Use a scale of 0 to 75, with:

$$0 = \text{No pain}$$
$$25 = \text{Mild pain}$$
$$50 = \text{Moderate pain}$$
$$75 = \text{Severe pain}$$

Judge the pain after each session and put the rating on your Daily Record. During the first week the values may be high, but by the second week you should begin to see the numbers heading toward 0. On day seven and fourteen, you will be graphing the week's pain ratings. The Pain Graph will give you a comprehensive picture of your progress.

The pain rating scale will be your best indicator of how effectively you are using the program. I will not remind you again about the scale, as it is your responsibility to rate the pain throughout the program. If you notice the rating is not decreasing enough, this may indicate that you need to practice additional Pain Control Imagery during the day, increasing from two minutes out of every waking hour to four or six minutes.

Daily Record

The Daily Record is to be copied into the pain control notebook and used twice each day. This serves as a constant reminder to perform the exercises and maintain a Daily Record of pain ratings.

A sample of the Daily Record for the first week is presented below and should serve as a model to copy from. Place an X in the appropriate box after completion of each assignment. Don't forget to rate your pain after each morning and evening session by placing a number—0, 25, 50, or 75—in the appropriate box, and to record your medication.

	DAY	1	2	3	4	5	6	7
MORNING	Exercises							
	Optional walk/run or exercycle							
	Pain Control Imagery							
	Pain Bonus							
	Record of Medication							
	Pain Rating							
EVENING	Exercises							
	Pain Control Imagery							
	Record of Medication							
	Pain Rating							

How to Make Your Pain Control Imagery Practice Tapes

Throughout my years of working with chronic pain patients and developing this program, I have tried constantly to design more effective ways to help patients practice on their own.

Initially, people came to my office for fifty-minute imagery sessions. There then might be a two- to three-day lapse before the next treatment. Practicing the Pain Control Imagery away from the clinic proved to be a worrisome, somewhat hit-or-miss affair for many patients. I also began to worry that others were becoming too dependent on me for treatment, rather than working at developing the skills for themselves.

Out of my concerns came the idea for taping Pain Control Imagery exercises. I began by taping them for patients, but I still was not totally satisfied with using my voice, since that placed patients in the position of receiving the therapy from an outside source rather than drawing on their own inner resources.

As a consequence, I decided to have each patient record the Pain Control Imagery exercises in his or her own voice (or that of a spouse or friend). By using this procedure, patients would be able to practice the exercises anywhere they could carry a tape recorder. By using their own voices they were completing the circle of responsibility for their own treatment process. After the basic approach was developed, we spent considerable time modifying the exercises for the self-treatment process. After many revisions, the Pain Control Imagery presented in this book is the refined, finished product.

NOTE: I strongly recommend that before you start the program you record all the Pain Control Imagery scripts to be used during the first week. You will find the scripts within the instructions for each day's exercises. Record all the scripts ahead of time and listen to the appropriate one each day.

TIPS ON MAKING YOUR OWN TAPES:

1. Carefully read over the complete script for each exercise before you record. The scripts are designed for direct reading into the tape recorder, so you should read them aloud several times before making the final recording.
2. Choose a spot and a time when you will have absolute quiet. Such distracting noises as a telephone ringing, a child yelling or a dog barking will interfere with your concentration when you listen to the tape.

3. Take your time! Read the sentences in a relaxed voice. Try to develop a rhythm in your speech. Do not rush!

Important Note:

When recording the instructions for tensing and relaxing the muscles, however, the tension exercises should be stated in an authoritative/demanding voice, while the instructions to relax should be in a soft, flowing, soothing tone.

4. Be careful not to speak too close to the microphone, for this may garble your voice and result in static. Run through a test session to see how far away from the mike you should speak.

5. After you have completed the tape, listen to it and compare it with the script.

6. If the tape is satisfactory, then punch out the tiny plastic tab at the back of the tape. When this is done, the tape cannot be recorded over by accident. The tab on the right is for side number one and the tab on the left is for side number two.

How to Start Each Pain Control Imagery Session

Each day the Pain Control Imagery session will be explained fully and the time needed to do it will be indicated. If your session runs fifteen minutes, then ask your family to allow you fifteen minutes of *uninterrupted practice time*. As you advance in the program, a quiet setting will not be quite so important, for you will learn how to complete the P.C.I. sessions even in the noisiest and most distracting situations.

Most people find the easiest posture for practicing is to lie flat on their backs. I recommend that you start out in this position, but hope that eventually you will be able to accomplish P.C.I. with your eyes open, in a sitting position, in a standing position or even while going about your daily activities. But for now, find a comfortable spot, whether the floor (some like the hard surface) or your bed, and stretch out. Do not cross your arms or legs. Your legs should be slightly apart with your hands to your sides, palms down. Place a pillow under your knees and one under your head. The pillow under the head is optional if you find that it's more comfortable to relax without it.

It would be nice if you could assume this position and immediately fall into a deeply relaxed state, but that is usually not the case; P.C.I., like any other technique, needs to be practiced often, and if you do, the successful control of pain is all yours. But don't try too hard. I have found that when you try to force relaxation, you get the opposite effect—tension.

Now that you've finished the preliminaries, let's get started with DAY ONE!

16

❧

Pain Control Program: Week One

TENSE/RELAX

Time: **40 Minutes Each Session**

TODAY'S ASSIGNMENT

Pain control begins with learning how to relax those tense, tight muscles. Also, I'll give you the secret to learning how to stop "thinking pain." Don't forget to copy the Daily Record into your notebook and check off each activity as you do it.

- Physical Reconditioning (twice)
- Pain Control Imagery: Relaxation Warm-Up and Script Number One—Tense/Relax (twice)
- Record Pain Level (twice)
- Pain Bonus: STOP THINKING PAIN (once)

PHYSICAL RECONDITIONING

Today marks the start of your exercise program. *Twice a day, every day* should be your bywords. Begin slowly on this first day. Here's the plan:

1. Head Rolls: two right, two left
2. Shoulders Up and Down: two
3. Arm Circles: two forward, two backward
4. Back Stretcher: two
5. Back Bender: two right, two left
6. Pelvic Tilt: twice
7. Single Knee to Chest: two each leg
8. Double Knee to Chest: two
9. Curl Downs: two
10. Curl Ups: two

Relaxation Warm-Up

Begin this exercise by assuming a comfortable position, preferably lying down. You may want to place a pillow under your knees to help the legs relax. Inhale deeply, and as you do, close your eyes and silently repeat the word "One" to yourself. Hold the breath for three seconds and then let it out very slowly, silently repeating the word "One" to yourself again. At the end of the exhalation, the abdomen should be moderately contracted. Repeat this procedure five times. Each time you breathe out, notice that there is a slight sag in your body. Your body will feel as though it is sinking down slightly. Let this happen; do not try to force anything. The relaxation warm-up is the preliminary exercise to start all the Pain Control Imagery sessions.

Now let's explore the quietness of your surroundings and become aware of any areas holding tension, especially pain sites.

Remember, you will never be able to get rid of absolutely all the tension in your body, as some levels are essential for maintaining attention, body structure and daily performance. I am mostly concerned with your learning how to get rid of the excess tension that feeds the fire of chronic pain.

Take a census of your muscle tension, starting at your feet and working up to the top of your head. Try to become aware of any muscles or groups of muscles that might be tense or hiding stress. As you reach your shoulders, pay close attention to the muscles of the back of your neck, the sides of your neck and your jaw.

Now take a deep breath and let your body sink down as you

exhale. Make sure that your arms are not touching the sides of your body and that your legs are slightly apart. Let your jaw sag and relax the muscles in your face.

You are going to be asked systematically to tense a specific muscle group and then hold it for at least three to five seconds and then relax, letting go of all the tightness and tension in that particular muscle.

> WARNING: DO NOT TENSE A MUSCLE TO THE POINT WHERE IT IS HURTING YOU. IF YOU HAVE HAD A BACK INJURY, NECK INJURY OR DAMAGE TO SOME SPECIFIC MUSCLE GROUP, THEN DO NOT TENSE THAT PARTICULAR MUSCLE AS MUCH AS THE OTHERS. BE AWARE OF YOUR OWN LIMITATIONS.

TURN ON THE TAPE RECORDER! Listen to Script Number One, which you have previously recorded.

Script Number One—Tense/Relax

Now it's time to begin. Allow yourself to find the most comfortable position you can. Make sure that none of your clothing is binding. If you have on a very tight wristwatch or ring, take it off. We do not want any extraneous sensations to interfere with your training procedure. Make sure that your head is supported so that it does not rock back and forth. Now take the deep breaths, letting them out slowly while you say the number "One" silently to yourself on the inhalation, and silently say the number "One" to yourself on the exhalation. Do this about five times and on the fifth time, allow your eyes to close.

Allow your thoughts to focus on your right hand. Form a mental picture of your hand and make a fist, squeezing tightly, holding the pressure for five to ten seconds. You may notice that your hand will tremble slightly; this is normal. Now let go. Let your fingers spread outward, letting all of the tension out. As you unclench your fist, you will notice that there are probably tingling sensations in your hand. This is the tension being released from the muscle. (Allow fifteen to twenty seconds to pass with your right hand in a relaxed position.) Study the difference between how your right hand felt when you were tensing it and how it now feels while you are relaxing. Make a fist again—hold it (five to ten seconds)—let go. Study the difference between tension and relaxation again. Allow this feeling of relaxation to become very familiar and notice how pleasing the sensation is when you let go.

Now visualize the muscles in your upper right arm, your biceps. Tense your biceps—hold it (five to ten seconds)—let go. Notice that your upper arm feels somewhat heavy and may even feel warm as you go deeper into body relaxation.

Now do the same with your left biceps. Tense them—hold it (five to ten seconds)—let go. Can you feel the tension flowing from your upper arms as you let go? Now tense all of the muscles in both of your arms—hold it (five to ten seconds)—let go.

Now we are going to tighten the muscles of the face. Lift your eyebrows as high as you can—hold it (five to ten seconds)—let go. Feel the tension flow from your forehead and scalp. Now do an exaggerated frown, bringing eyebrows together—hold it (five to ten seconds)—let go.

Close your eyes tightly and wrinkle your nose—hold it (five to ten seconds)—let go. Feel the tension in the upper part of your cheeks and around your eyes flow out of your body.

Clench your teeth together and pull the corners of your mouth back as if brushing your teeth—hold it (five to ten seconds)—let go. Feel the tension flowing from your lower face and jaw.

Try to push your chin down toward your chest while trying to pull your head back in the opposite direction, pitting one set of muscles against the other—hold it (five to ten seconds)—let go. Notice that there might be a slight tremor of tension as the opposing muscles begin to release their tension.

Take a deep breath and hold it and at the same time bring your shoulder blades together, bringing them back as if to touch them—hold it (five to ten seconds)—let go. Feel the tension in the chest, back and upper back release as you let go.

Tightly arch your lower back away from the back of the chair—hold it (five to ten seconds)—let go. Feel the tension in the two rows of muscles running alongside of the spine release all of their stored pain and tightness.

Tighten your stomach muscles as if you were warding off a

blow—hold it (five to ten seconds)—let go. The abdomen may feel slightly tense afterward and gradually you'll notice it beginning to relax.

Tighten your upper legs (thighs) by trying to push your knees together and apart at the same time. While doing this, try to push your legs down and lift them up at the same time—hold it (five to ten seconds)—let go. Your upper leg muscles have gotten harder, but notice the tension flowing from them.

Carefully pull your toes up toward your head (care should be taken so as not to cramp the calf muscles)—hold it (five to ten seconds)—let go. The calf muscles will remain tight for several seconds but then you'll feel the relaxing warmth flowing into them.

Curl your feet and toes as if you were making a fist (don't tighten too hard in order to prevent cramping)—hold it (five to ten seconds)—let go. Feel the tension flowing from your feet. Study the relaxation, and notice the difference between tension and relaxation in the muscles of your toes and your feet. Maintain relaxation in your calves and thighs while you are working with your feet. Now try it again, tensing the muscles in your toes and feet. Maintain relaxation in your calves and thighs while you are working with your feet. Now try it again, tensing the muscles in your toes and feet—hold it (five to ten seconds)—let go. Now it is time to check for any areas of tension in your body. Start at your toes while you are maintaining a deep relaxation and run a check up your body through all the muscles with which we have worked. Check on some muscles that we have not talked about, and if you find them tense, try the tense/relax exercise and you will find that even the most tense muscle can become relaxed. While you are relaxing, remember that your lips should be slightly parted and you should maintain that smooth, rhythmical breathing. Allow the warm, heavy feeling to flow throughout your body, reaching deep into the muscles.

Spend the next five minutes remaining in this position and tensing and relaxing any of the muscles at will. Try for the deepest state of relaxation possible, while studying the difference between tension and relaxation.

When you are ready to terminate the exercise, simply:

· *Make the decision to stop*
· *Flex your arms*
· *Flex your legs*
· *Take a deep breath*
· *Open your eyes.*

A Word of Caution:

When you finish any of the relaxation exercises, sit up slowly, allowing yourself to stretch. If you sit up too quickly, you can become hypotensive and experience some dizziness. If you should feel dizzy, lie down again and stretch the muscles in your arms and legs, sitting up more slowly the next time.

This tape should be listened to at least twice during the first day. If you have time, additional practice periods would be extremely beneficial.

Don't forget to note your Pain Level in your Daily Record.

PAIN BONUS: STOP THINKING PAIN

It is understandable that anyone who is in pain thinks about it most of the time. But there are two ways to be preoccupied with your pain; one is negative, the other positive.

Negative Preoccupation

You can't seem to get your mind off the pain and when you do become distracted for a few moments, it may be to think about someone else's pain or problems. There seems to be a never ending parade of thoughts centered around your suffering. You find discussions with your family and friends are almost always centered on your pain and you may even find that some friends are not coming around quite so often since you've been preoccupied with your pain. Your negative thoughts are a circular track and the pain train chugs round and round.

Positive Thoughts

No one is asking you to pretend that your pain is not there, but I am asking you to turn your negative pain thoughts into positive ones. Here are a few examples:

- You can control your pain.
- You are becoming more active.
- You are constantly moving forward.
- Pain Control Imagery is a key to a whole new way of life.
- Positive thinking is contagious.

USING PAIN THOUGHT STOPPING

Pain thought stopping is a very simple, yet extremely effective technique that you can use to stop the anticipation of pain and allow Pain Control Imagery to work more effectively. The technique works on the principle that you cannot think about two things at once; your body cannot be both tense and relaxed at the same time. You should use this technique only on chronic pain. You should not use Pain Thought Stopping to block the body's warning signals (pain) relating to a new discomfort that has not been evaluated by your physician.

Pain Thought Stopping (P.T.S.) needs to be practiced on a daily basis. In the beginning you will have to make a conscious effort to go through the exercise, but after a short period of time, the P.T.S. will activate automatically, thus short-circuiting the fear and anticipation of pain and allowing you to activate the built-in painkiller whenever needed.

Objectives
1. To stop anticipatory pain.
2. To interfere with the pain response.
3. To allow the Pain Control Imagery to signal the release of endorphin.

Read through the simple steps I have listed for you and practice your Pain Thought Stopping EVERY time you find yourself thinking negative thoughts.

Step One:
Close your eyes and begin thinking about your pain. When you have these pain thoughts firmly in your mind, yell the word, "Stop!" as loudly as you can. You will notice that the

word "Stop" immediately interrupts your thought process. Follow the word "Stop" with a deep breath, and as you breathe in, repeat silently to yourself the words "I am," and as you breathe out, say the word "Relaxed." Perform the "I am relaxed" technique with five deep breaths.

Step Two:

Since it is not socially acceptable to yell "STOP" in public, you will have to practice the exercise using a "mental STOP" which will entail your simply saying to yourself mentally, "Stop." A practice aid I have found very effective is to place a rubber band around your wrist and as you mentally say "Stop," snap the rubber band against your wrist, thus serving as a reinforcement. Always remember to perform the "I AM RELAXED" exercise immediately following the "Stop."

Step Three:

In the beginning this exercise may seem quite cumbersome, but after practicing it, the reaction will become nearly automatic. Of course, this form of negative thought stopping can be used for any negative thoughts that might interfere with positive thinking.

Step Four:

In order to become effective, thought stopping needs to be practiced many times during the day. Your goal is to establish it as an automatic response.

PAIN THOUGHT STOPPING FORMULA

When the four steps of Pain Thought Stopping are combined, you have the perfect formula for breaking the bad habit of always thinking of pain. Copy the formula into your notebook and use it often. Developing P.T.S. will be an effective tool you can use to reduce pain.

THOUGHTS OF PAIN → (Activates) → P.T.S. → (Leads To) → PAIN REDUCTION

SELF-HYPNOSIS

Time: **45 Minutes Each Session**

TODAY'S ASSIGNMENT

After mastering the basics of relaxation, the next step is to reach your innermost controls. Keep your spirits up as I show you how to stop "Pain Talk."

- Physical Reconditioning (twice)
- Pain Control Imagery: Script Number Two—Self-Hypnosis (twice)
- Record Pain Level (twice)
- Pain Bonus: Pain Talk (once)

PHYSICAL RECONDITIONING

1. Head Rolls: two right, two left
2. Shoulders Up and Down: Four
3. Arm Circles: four forward, four backward
4. Back Stretcher: four
5. Back Bender: two right, two left
6. Pelvic Tilt: two
7. Single Knee to Chest: four each leg
8. Double Knee to Chest: four
9. Curl Downs: four
10. Curl Ups: four

PAIN CONTROL IMAGERY

In today's session you will be introduced to the first steps of learning self-hypnosis, combined with some mental imagery. This will be an exciting session and you will find that the amount of relaxation achieved will be much greater than with progressive relaxation.

You should listen to this session once in the morning and once in the evening, but that's only a minimum; it would be better for you to listen more times during the day. Practice parts of the session on your own without the tape and see if you can achieve the same results.

NOTE: Don't forget the relaxation warm-up before the Pain Control Imagery. (See p. 170.)

TURN ON THE TAPE RECORDER

Script Number Two—Self-Hypnosis

Assume a comfortable position.
Take a deep breath and let it out slowly.
Close your eyes.
Let's begin.
Lie back comfortably in the chair.
Let yourself go . . . loose, limp and slack.
Let all the muscles of your body relax completely.
Breathe in and out . . . nice and slow.
Concentrate on your feet and ankles and let them relax.
Let them relax . . . let them go . . . loose, limp and slack.
Soon you will begin to feel a feeling of heaviness in your feet.
Your feet are beginning to feel as heavy as lead.
Your feet are getting heavier and heavier.
Let yourself go completely.
Now let all of the muscles of your calves and thighs go loose, limp and slack.
Let all of these muscles in your legs relax totally and completely.
Your legs are beginning to feel heavier and heavier.
Let yourself go completely.
Give yourself up totally to this very pleasant . . . relaxed . . . comfortable feeling.
Let your whole body go loose, limp and slack.
Your whole body is becoming as heavy as lead.
Let the muscles of your stomach completely relax.
Let them become loose, limp and slack.

Next the muscles of your chest and your back.

Let them go completely loose, limp and slack, and as you feel heaviness in your body, you are relaxing more deeply.

Your whole body is becoming just as heavy as lead.

Let yourself sink down deeper in the chair.

Let yourself relax totally and completely.

Let all of the muscles in your neck and shoulders relax.

Let all of these muscles go loose, limp and slack.

Now the muscles in your arms are becoming loose, limp, slack and heavy.

As they relax, they are getting heavier and heavier.

As though your arms are as heavy as lead.

Let your arms go.

Let your whole body relax completely.

Your whole body is deeply and completely relaxed.

Now a feeling of complete relaxation is gradually moving over your whole body.

All of the muscles in your feet and ankles are completely relaxed.

Your calf and thigh muscles are completely relaxed.

All of the muscles in your legs are loose, limp and slack.

And as you relax . . . your sleep is becoming deeper and more relaxing.

The feeling of relaxation is spreading through all of your body.

All of the muscles of your body are becoming loose, limp and slack.

Totally relaxed.

Your body is getting heavier and heavier.

You are going deeper and deeper into relaxation.

As your relaxation increases . . . your pain is becoming less and less.

Endorphins are moving to the sites of pain in your body.

You are becoming so completely relaxed and comfortable that the pain is disappearing completely.

From this time on, you will be able to give yourself a treatment.

Any time, any place, any where.

Whenever you want to give yourself a treatment.

All you will have to do is count from twenty to one.

Count slowly and feel yourself sinking down into a deep relaxation.

When you are totally relaxed, you will be able to give yourself any suggestions you desire regarding pain.

You will be able to activate your body's built-in painkiller.

If any unexpected emergency should arise during your deep sleep, you will automatically wake up and take any necessary action.

When you have given yourself suggestions, you may wake yourself up.

Slowly count from one to five and when you say the number five to yourself, your eyes will open and you will be wide awake.

Flex your arms and legs and sit up slowly.

Just like riding a bicycle, proper training in self-hypnosis takes practice and perseverance. Self-hypnosis will serve as a stepping stone to the pain imagery formulas you will be learning during the second week of the Program.

RECORD PAIN LEVEL IN YOUR DAILY RECORD

Each time you practice your P.C.I. or exercises, don't forget to note them in your Daily Record, along with comments or reminders to yourself. Your personal comments are very important, for they serve as progress hints. It is possible to forget from one day to the next which exercise provided you the most relief or presented the greatest problem.

PAIN BONUS: PAIN TALK

Constant talking about your pain is strictly forbidden in the Pain Control Program!

You must always remember: if you focus on your suffering, your suffering probably will increase; whereas, if you focus on pain control, the chances are great that you will be able to decrease the pain.

Some of the negative consequences of "pain talk" are chronicled below.

Helen spent at least four hours a day talking on the phone with her friends in long, involved sessions that centered on the comparison of operations, aches and pains, and future pain. After the morning session of phone calls, Helen was exhausted and would lie down for the rest of the day, depressed and feeling more pain.

Learning to Stop the Pain Talk

Now is the time to break the habit of pain talk, and I'll show you how you can accomplish this.

Before I list the ways to break the pain talk habit, take a few minutes and turn to a blank page in your pain control notebook. Jot down the times when you seem to talk most about the pain. Is it when you're with your neighbor? When you're with your spouse? When you're under stress? Early in the morning? Try to find when exactly you do most of your pain talk.

Just to make sure you have pinpointed all the pain talk, ask your spouse or someone close to you if they know of any times when you seem to always talk about your pain.

The most difficult time in breaking the pain talk habit will be in the beginning. If you've ever tried to stop smoking, lose weight or change any bad habit, you'll realize the most difficult part is starting and that is why I've provided you with these tips.

Tip 1: Go Cold Turkey.

Stop the pain talk right now! Don't figure that you can taper off slowly. Even using pain talk a few times during the day reinforces the behavior.

Tip 2: Don't Give In!

Don't forget to reward yourself for not talking about your pain. If there is a favorite television program, a movie you've wanted to see or some other type of positive reward, use it to reinforce non–pain talk behavior.

A little warning: don't use reinforcers such as eating, smoking or drinking as rewards. You may develop an equally bad habit. Turn the page in your pain control notebook and list five rewards. Use one reward for each of the first five days of the program. Do not make the rewards too grandiose, but small enough that they can be used at the end of the day. Put some time and thought into this, and list as your sixth reward a fairly large one that can be used over the weekend if you have been successful each of the previous five days. At the beginning of the next week, make a similar list with a larger reward for that weekend. By the end of the second week your pain talk behavior should be nonexistent, but this should not prevent you from continuing your vigil against it. Of course, your greatest reward will come at the end of the program and that will be freedom from pain.

Tip 3: Forgetting the Mistakes.

If you should make a mistake and talk about your pain—and chances are you will at some point early in your program—don't fret over your lapse. Try to figure out what went wrong, what keyed your break in behavior. When you realize where the mistake lies, prevent it from happening again.

Spending all of your time beating yourself with a mental bat is not the way to correct a flaw. Analyze the mistake, resolve not to make the same mistake again, and move forward with your program.

AUTOGENICS

Time: 35 Minutes Each Session

TODAY'S ASSIGNMENT

You're into the third day of the program, and it's time for me to teach you the third segment of self-control. So far, I've concentrated on methods that are long and involved. Autogenics is short, quick and to the point—pain control. I've always found the guilt of pain to be destructive, so I am providing you a method to overcome it.

- Physical Reconditioning (twice)
- Pain Control Imagery: Script Number Three—Autogenics (twice)
- Record Pain Level (twice)
- Pain Bonus: The Guilt of Pain (once)

PHYSICAL RECONDITIONING

At this point in the exercise program you will be noticing some soreness from muscles that may not have been used for a long time. Muscle soreness at the start of exercising may cause some people to stop. Don't stop. It may take up to a week for tight muscles to stretch out; then "good-bye, soreness!"

1. Head Rolls: two right, two left
2. Shoulders Up and Down: four
3. Arm Circles: six forward, six backward
4. Back Stretcher: six
5. Back Bender: two right, two left
6. Pelvic Tilt: four
7. Single Knee to Chest: five each leg

8. Double Knee to Chest: five
9. Curl Downs: four
10. Curl Ups: four

Pain Control Imagery

Today you will be beginning the autogenics phase of Pain Control Imagery. During the previous two days, you should have learned the basics of the tense/relax and the beginnings of basic self-hypnosis. You should, of course, review these at various times during the program.

Learning autogenic training as your first step toward mental imagery and activating your built-in painkiller system is a very needed task. As you begin to use the autogenic formula, you may notice that certain variations work better than others and some alterations may need to be made. This is why I have compiled the list of tips to help you learn autogenics faster and more effectively.

Autogenic Tips:
1. Whenever an exercise formula calls for warmth and you feel too warm, change the formula to "slightly warm."
2. If warmth seems to bother you, then you may change the formula to "coolness."
3. Whenever using "coolness" around the forehead or face, you may want to use the words "slightly cool." Some people who have visualized ice on their faces develop an ice-cream headache (see Mini Dictionary of Pain). Using the word "slightly" to modify either coolness or warmth is appropriate.
4. In the beginning stages of autogenic training, there is usually some twitching of muscles; this is simply a nervous discharge as you go deeper into relaxation. If you don't worry about it, it will gradually disappear.
5. Whenever repeating the phrases regarding a specific area of the body, try to visualize that area in your mind's eye. This helps train you to focus on different body areas and will be used later to activate the endorphins to specific areas.

6. Never sit up quickly after the end of an exercise, for this may cause you to become hypotensive and develop dizziness and possibly faint.

7. Please remember that any modification of the formula should be done very carefully and thought out first. The main guide in any modification should be *common sense*.

Practice Schedule

The tape of this session should be listened to at least twice daily. Once in the morning and once in the evening is sufficient, but real benefits can come from your practicing the phrases on your own at other times during the day. In order to practice some of the phrases, copy them into your notebook, or carry a listing with you. Between the morning and evening session, silently repeat the phrases to yourself every chance you have.

Don't forget the warm-up relaxation exercise described on page 170. Do it before listening to the autogenics tape.

TURN ON THE TAPE RECORDER.

Script Number Three—Autogenics

Clear all extraneous thoughts from your mind by counting from ten to one silently to yourself. Picture each number in your mind's eye as you count down, and when you reach the number one, take a deep breath and let it out slowly.

I want you to repeat each one of the phrases five times, silently to yourself, as I present them to you. There should be a five-second interval between each phrase. This will allow you the time to repeat to yourself. Picture in your mind that part of the body which we are talking about. As you repeat each phrase, do so in a rhythmic manner. Try to maintain normal, even breathing.

Take a deep breath.

Let it out . . . slowly.

Close . . . your eyes.

(*Ten seconds*)

My right arm . . . is heavy.
(Five seconds between phrases . . . repeat five times.)

My left arm . . . is heavy.
(Five seconds between phrases . . . repeat five times.)

My arms . . . are heavy.
(Five seconds between phrases . . . repeat five times.)

My left leg . . . is heavy.
(Five seconds between phrases . . . repeat five times.)

My right leg . . . is heavy.
(Five seconds between phrases . . . repeat five times.)

My legs . . . are heavy.
(Five seconds between phrases . . . repeat five times.)

My right arm . . . is warm.
(Five seconds between phrases . . . repeat five times.)

My left arm . . . is warm.
(Five seconds between phrases . . . repeat five times.)

My arms . . . are warm.
(Five seconds between phrases . . . repeat five times.)

My right leg . . . is warm.
(Five seconds between phrases . . . repeat five times.)

My left leg . . . is warm.
(Five seconds between phrases . . . repeat five times.)

My legs . . . are warm.
(Five seconds between phrases . . . repeat five times.)

My heartbeat . . . is calm and regular.
(Five seconds between phrases . . . repeat five times.)

My breathing . . . is calm and regular.
(Five seconds between phrases . . . repeat five times.)

My stomach . . . is warm.
(Five seconds between phrases . . . repeat five times.)

My forehead . . . is cool.
(Five seconds between phrases . . . repeat five times.)

I am . . . at peace.
(Five seconds between phrases . . . repeat five times.)

I am . . . relaxed.
(Five seconds between phrases . . . repeat five times.)

RECORD PAIN LEVEL IN YOUR DAILY RECORD

PAIN BONUS: THE GUILT OF PAIN

"God must be punishing me."
"I feel so guilty that my family has suffered from my pain."
"I feel guilty about eating, so I eat more."
"Our savings have been destroyed by my pain."
"I've been a burden on everyone."

Guilty by Reason of Pain

Guilt is a definite part of any pain problem. When you experience discomfort constantly, other members of your family, friends and associates at work will be affected by your pain. A coworker might have to take over an extra load, your spouse may have to find a job or an extra job to help supplement the family income, a son or daughter might not be able to get a new bike this year because the money has to be used to pay medical bills.

Guilt is a common symptom of any prolonged pain condition. Society tells us that it is okay to feel guilty when you've suffered from chronic pain, and, in fact, it appears to be an expected behavior.

CASE

David B. hurt his neck in an automobile accident and, after several futile attempts at returning to work and unsuccessful therapy, which included acupuncture, alcohol, nerve blocks and physical therapy, he was no longer able to maintain his job. His wife was agreeable to the idea of working at a part-time job and Dave tried to help out with as much of the housework as possible. Even pushing the vacuum cleaner made the pain unbearable, so the young children took over most of the housework. Most of his mornings were spent in bed, watching but not seeing an endless parade of quiz shows and soap operas. He was overcome with guilt about causing the family hardship. He also felt guilt about the children, especially his ten-year-old son. On weekends, David would lie on the couch, looking out the window as his wife threw a football with his son.

When I talked with Dave, he told me, "I don't feel like a man. I feel guilty about everything."

Something had to be done. David's guilt added to his suffering and was preventing him from reducing pain.

Here are the action steps I gave to Dave. They can help you, too!

Step One:
Sit down with your family and explain to them how you feel. Be honest and open about your emotions and ask them for their feelings.

Step Two:
With your family, draw up a list of responsibilities you can still accomplish. This is, a process of redefining your role within the family unit. All members of the family should realize that their roles are constantly changing throughout life and your role will definitely change as you experience a reduction in your pain.

Step Three:
Plan a weekly meeting, at a specific time and on a specific day. All family members should discuss their feelings and ideas at this meeting. Increased communication among family members will help you to fight the effects of guilt.

Try to keep in mind that guilt is not an outside "invader," but something which develops from within. You have to make the decision not to be guilty, and good communication is the best medicine.

AUTOGENICS REPEAT

Time: **35 Minutes Each Session**

TODAY'S ASSIGNMENT

Yesterday's Pain Control Imagery was only the first step. The secret to autogenics' success is constant repetition. If learning pain control is really what you want, then take some time out of your busy day to practice autogenics.

- Physical Reconditioning (twice)
- Pain Control Imagery: Repeat Tape Number Three— Autogenics (twice)
- Record Pain Level (twice)
- Pain Bonus: Pain as an Escape (once)

PHYSICAL RECONDITIONING

Spend some time taking a walk today. Get out and stretch your legs. Consider the optional walk/run program.

1. Head Rolls: three right, three left
2. Shoulders Up and Down: five
3. Arm Circles: six forward, six backward
4. Back Stretcher: six
5. Back Bender: three right, three left
6. Pelvic Tilt: four
7. Single Knee to Chest: six each leg
8. Double Knee to Chest: six
9. Curl Downs: four
10. Curl Ups: four

PAIN CONTROL IMAGERY

Today's assignment will be to listen to the autogenic training tape of Day Three once in the morning and once in the evening. Don't forget to practice during the day by using the autogenic phrases you copied into your notebook. The warm, relaxed feeling you will obtain through using the autogenic exercises will definitely begin to reduce the amount of pain caused by muscular tension. Before listening to the tape, don't forget the relaxation warm-up on page 170.

NOTE: You may practice the autogenic exercises with your eyes open if you prefer. Some people even practice these exercises while doing their exercises or optional walk/run.

PAIN BONUS: PAIN AS AN ESCAPE

Pain can be used as a form of escape, an excuse or alibi for not doing something. The escape mechanism of pain can work on a conscious or unconscious level, but the end result is the same: when you're in pain you're not expected to become involved in certain activities or perform certain tasks.

CASE

Every time Doris P. is on a date, she notices an increase in her tension headaches. Whenever her date makes any sexual advances toward her, she feels the pain increasing in the back of her neck and head. Even thinking about a date causes her to perspire, tremble and experience a tension headache. As a young girl she had some bad experiences in dating situations and on one occasion had a headache that allowed her to cancel the date. Very soon a pattern of behavior was established using the headache as an excuse to avoid the anxiety of dating.

CASE

Mike had a hard day at work and as he drove home, thoughts of mowing the lawn, finishing the carpentry in his daughter's room, the cries for help with homework ran through his mind. By the time he pulled into the driveway,

Mike had the beginning of a headache. As he entered the house and said to his wife, "Boy, it's been a hard day. I've really got a headache," she followed with, "Poor dear, let me get you some aspirin and you can rest." She turned to the children. "Your father has had a very hard day and has a headache. Don't bother him now." The children are shuffled off to another part of the house and pampering of the headachy husband begins. Mike is allowed to rest undisturbed for an hour and at the end of that time, his headache is gone.

Mike has discovered a manipulative behavior and each time he complains of a headache, the family reacts in a specific manner. Mike has received a payoff from his pain and the cycle is set.

Check to make sure that you are not using pain as an escape. No matter how fast you run or how far you travel, the pain will stay with you until resolved.

THE INWARD JOURNEY

Time: 25 Minutes Each Session

TODAY'S ASSIGNMENT

Exciting is the word to describe today's activity.

· Physical Reconditioning (twice)
· Pain Control Imagery: Script Number Four—The Inward Journey (twice)
· Record Pain Level (twice)
· Pain Bonus: Sexual Activity and Pain (once)

PHYSICAL RECONDITIONING

1. Head Rolls: four right, four left
2. Shoulders Up and Down: six
3. Arm Circles: six forward, six backward
4. Back Stretcher: eight
5. Back Bender: four right, four left
6. Pelvic Tilt: four
7. Single Knee to Chest: six each leg
8. Double Knee to Chest: six
9. Curl Downs: five
10. Curl Ups: five

PAIN CONTROL IMAGERY

Today we're going to embark upon a journey inside your body through the use of Pain Control Imagery. This will be your first session designed to help you specifically activate the body's built-in painkiller—ENDORPHINS.

This exercise should be performed twice daily.

Remember: You should be practicing your autogenics

throughout the day. And do your relaxation warm-up (page 170) before beginning this tape.

TURN TAPE RECORDER ON.

Script Number Four—The Inward Journey

Let's go to work.
Take a deep breath.
Let it out slowly.
Close your eyes.
My arms and legs are heavy and warm.
My heartbeat is calm and regular.
My breathing is calm and regular.
My stomach is warm.
My forehead is cool.

(Stop repeating the phrases!
You are ready to begin *THE INWARD JOURNEY*.)

As I continue to feel this deep inward calmness, I focus my attention on my breathing. I sense the cool air coming into my lungs as I breathe in, and I feel the warmth of my breath as I exhale. As I experience the calm, deeply relaxed sensations of my breathing, I visualize oxygen traveling down into my body, down into my lungs, picture an oxygen molecule going deeper and deeper into my lungs. Finally, I can see the oxygen molecule arriving in my lungs and I begin to hear the sound of my blood rushing into my lungs and becoming louder and louder as it approaches the place to pick up the oxygen molecule. I now see the blood rushing past the molecule of oxygen, picking it up and carrying it up my chest, up further and further, into my neck, past my neck, toward my brain. I picture my brain slowly coming into view—a grayish mass of tissue with tiny sparks of electricity as the oxygen molecule is carried by the blood closer and closer to my brain. I can see and hear the sound of my brain working as the blood—my blood—carries this oxygen molecule into my brain to be used as energy. I can see the oxygen being taken up from the bloodstream by my brain and being burned up as energy. As this oxygen is being used, I can see another substance being formed, another substance made possible by the brain—my brain—using the oxygen as energy. At first I can see this new substance slowly being produced as the oxygen is slowly burned. I can see clearly now that this substance is a painkilling substance called endorphin. I can see these painkilling substances beginning to flow through my brain as more and more are produced. As more and more of these painkilling substances called endorphins are produced, I can feel them beginning to spread outside my brain, beginning to spread throughout my body, bringing comfort and relief as they do their job. I can now feel these endorphins, these painkilling substances, spreading down my neck, down into the area of my chest and upper arms. I enjoy the comfort, the soothing sensation that these endorphins bring. I can now feel these endorphins spreading more and more into my lower arms, my hands, my lower back and stomach. Gradually I feel these painkilling substances spreading down into my upper and lower legs and finally into my feet, bringing comfort, relief, a soothing sensation as they continue to reduce my level of discomfort. I can now visualize quite clearly these helpful, painkilling substances spreading more and more throughout my whole body.

I sense my body becoming normal, functioning completely, healthily, comfortably, and pain-free.

All of my body and mind are functioning together to block pain.

I see and feel my body and mind learning to block the pain response.

I feel and experience a quiet, deep comfort, knowing that my body and mind are working together to help my body.

I feel a new energy flowing through my legs, hips and back.

I feel a new energy flowing through my stomach, chest and arms.

I feel a new energy flowing through my neck, head and face. The energy makes me feel good.

I open my eyes, flex my arms and legs, and feel wide awake.

NOTE: Turn off the recorder.

Now wasn't that a great session?

RECORD PAIN LEVEL IN YOUR DAILY RECORD.
PAIN BONUS: SEXUAL ACTIVITY AND PAIN

"Not tonight, I've got a headache!"

"My back hurts too much!"

"When I'm in pain, I can't do anything!"

"I just don't seem to be interested . . . or have the urge."

Discounting those who invent pain or develop imaginary headaches as an excuse to avoid sexual activity, people who suffer from pain do have particular problems regarding sexual activity. Back injuries are the worst culprits.

CASE

Dennis suffered a back injury three years ago and after several operations and numerous treatments ranging from physical therapy to acupuncture, he still had at least 30 percent of his discomfort. He was able to return to work and he maintained full-time employment, but his marital relationship was on a downward slide. During his recoveries from surgery, intercourse with his wife was totally forbidden and they accepted it as a fact of life and looked forward to the time when they could resume their sexual intimacy. After an okay from the surgeon, Dennis and his wife resumed intercourse and from the very first time, he experienced pain during the act and increasing discomfort following it. His wife noticed the decrease in their sexual activity and wondered if she was becoming less attractive. He reassured her that that was not the case but never admitted his worries regarding reinjury and increased pain. Intercourse became less frequent, and each time he thought about performing the sexual act his level of anxiety increased and so did his stress. Now he was faced with an additional problem: impotence. The anticipation of pain and the worry over reinjury were causing him to become impotent, adding to his worries.

Dennis's problems are faced by millions of men and women who have suffered injuries and experience pain during sexual acts. I sat down with Dennis and his wife to explain how this problem could be stopped and further troubles avoided.

Here is what I advised Dennis and his wife:

- Avoid intercourse during times of peak pain.
- The partner with the back problem should be in the underneath position with a pillow placed under the buttocks to elevate the hips.
- Intercourse while lying on your side with the knees bent may prevent pain from pelvic contortions.
- Stay away from gymnastic positions.
- Lead up to the sexual act gradually, taking full advantage of massage techniques.

An excellent book is *The Joy of Sex* by Alex Comfort, published by Simon & Schuster, which illustrates a variety of positions and sexual techniques. If you have a particular question regarding one of the techniques, consult your family physician.

THERAPY THOUGHT: *The key to sexual activity during painful states is twofold: good communication between partners and a willingness to learn comfortable positions.*

PAIN STICKERS

Time: **20 Minutes Each Session**

TODAY'S ASSIGNMENT

Pain stickers will always keep you on your toes. Once you learn to use the stickers, pain control will be as automatic as breathing.

- Physical Reconditioning (twice)
- Troubleshooting Your P.C.I. (once)
- Pain Control Imagery: Pain Stickers (twice)
- Pain Bonus: Pain Popsicle (as needed)

PHYSICAL RECONDITIONING

Take a few minutes to review the exercises in Chapter Fourteen to insure that you are performing each exercise properly.

1. Head Rolls: four right, four left
2. Shoulders Up and Down: eight
3. Arm Circles: eight forward, eight backward
4. Back Stretcher: eight
5. Back Bender: eight right, eight left
6. Pelvic Tilt: four
7. Single Knee to Chest: six each leg
8. Double Knee to Chest: six
9. Curl Downs: six
10. Curl Ups: six

TROUBLESHOOTING
YOUR PAIN CONTROL IMAGERY

During the course of Pain Control Imagery, problems may develop. Here are some solutions.

1. Cramps in certain muscles. You may be tensing too hard. Ease up on your tension for that particular muscle group.
2. Spasms and twitches may be expected, especially if you have been a very up-tight person for most of your life. The more you focus on them, the more frequent they become. Many of us experience spasms at night after falling asleep but are not aware of them.
3. Coughing and sneezing. Bring yourself out of the relaxation and try again. Don't try to stop yourself from sneezing. If you must, go ahead and sneeze, but then go back into the relaxation.
4. You may experience some strange sensations such as heaviness or lightness, coolness or warmth during your first stages of relaxation. Don't let them bother you; your body is adjusting to a new form of functioning (relaxation). Some people even experience a sensation of floating during the relaxation and this is very beneficial. Floating or dis-associated feelings are indicative of deep relaxation.
5. Increased sexual arousal. Sometimes during a deep state of relaxation, sexual arousal may occur. It does not signify a problem.
6. Sometimes when a person is in a deep state of relaxation, he or she has the sensation of losing control. I reassure you that you will not lose control, since you are doing the talking on the tape and the relaxation is totally safe.

Your Goal

Your goal for Pain Control Imagery will be to attain total body relaxation within twenty seconds and be able to maintain that relaxation for two minutes. When relaxation is achieved this quickly, it can be used to preempt the pain response before it gets started.

PAIN STICKERS

The reprograming of your body's response to pain continues.

For this exercise you'll need either masking tape or small colored adhesive disks, which can be purchased at any stationery store. Place a sticker on areas such as: the top of your car steering wheel, the crystal of your watch, the refrigerator door, your telephone, your desk and any other place you frequent during the day. The stickers will be your special reminders.

Whenever you see a reminder sticker during the day, this exercise should be repeated once. For your longer morning and evening sessions, please tape this exercise running through the entire sequence five times (approximately twenty to thirty minutes).

Do your relaxation warm-up and then TURN ON THE TAPE RECORDER.

Script Number Five—Pain Stickers

1. *Take a deep breath.*
2. *Let it out slowly.*
3. *Let your body relax totally.*
4. *Repeat each phrase below five times silently to yourself.*

I can block my pain.
My arms and legs are heavy and warm.
My heartbeat is calm and regular.
My breathing is calm and regular.
My stomach is warm.
My forehead is cool.
Take a deep breath.
Flex your arms and legs.
Awake, refreshed and totally relaxed!

At this point in the program, it should be quite clear that I'm flooding you with Pain Control Imagery. This flooding builds and reinforces pain control.

RECORD YOUR PAIN LEVEL.

PAIN BONUS: PAIN POPSICLE

I must warn you before we start that ice massages may not be one of the more pleasant techniques in this book, but could possibly be one of the most effective for neck and back pain.

Almost everyone is familiar with the use of heat to help ease aching, painful muscles and joints, and most likely at some time during your life you've taken a hot bath or shower to ease the aches and pains of your back and neck. In some cases heat is an effective method for dilating (opening) the blood vessels and increasing the amount of painful lactates that are carried away from the site of discomfort. Unfortunately, heat has several drawbacks: heat (even damp heat) does not penetrate very deep below the skin, and heat may cause an increase in hemorrhaging (bleeding) of an injury.

Ice does not have the two major drawbacks of heat and it penetrates two to three times deeper than heat, constricts (makes smaller) the blood vessels and thereby decreases the chance of internal bleeding, and slows and retards the transmission of pain impulses along the nerve pathways. Ice massage can also be used as often as needed with no harmful side effects.

Ice massage may not help rid everyone of discomfort, but patients have found it useful for: back pain, neck pain, painful joints (elbow, knees) and muscle strains.

Since ice massage may be uncomfortable when you first start it, a short period of time should be allowed for adjustment to the technique.

Making Your Pain Popsicle

Making your pain popsicle is just about as easy as using it.

Step One: Take several Styrofoam cups and fill them with water to within one-half inch of the top.

Step Two: Place the cups of water in the freezer for at least four to six hours.

Step Three: Remove a cup as needed and with a table knife, score a line around the cup one inch from the top. You will be able to peel off this top section, leaving the bottom part of the cup for you to grasp with half an inch of ice exposed at the top. As the ice is used in massage, the Styrofoam may be gradually cut until you need a new cup.

Step Four: When the ice is first applied to the skin, there is an expected uncomfortable sensation. Don't let this stop you, but do your relaxation while the ice massage is being applied and, believe it or not, after a period of time you will become accustomed to the ice.

Step Five: Doing it yourself or having someone do it for you, move the ice in either a circular or back-and-forth motion across the area of discomfort. Keep the ice in contact with the skin and use a towel to catch any excess water.

Step Six: Do not use the massage for more than two to three minutes at a time. The procedure may be repeated as needed.

INTERNAL PAIN BLOCK

Time: 20 Minutes Each Session

TODAY'S ASSIGNMENT

Congratulations are in order. You've finished the first week!

- Physical Reconditioning (twice)
- Pain Control Imagery: Internal Pain Block (twice)
- Record Pain Level (twice)
- Pain Bonus: Leisure Activities (once)
- Pain Graph (once)
- Personal Pain Diagram

PHYSICAL RECONDITIONING

1. Head Rolls: four right, four left
2. Shoulders Up and Down: ten
3. Arm Circles: ten forward, ten backward
4. Back Stretcher: ten
5. Back Bender: eight right, eight left
6. Pelvic Tilt: four
7. Single Knee to Chest: eight each leg
8. Double Knee to Chest: eight
9. Curls Downs: six
10. Curl Ups: six

PAIN CONTROL IMAGERY:
INTERNAL PAIN BLOCK

Up until this point you've learned progressive relaxation, self-hypnosis, autogenic therapy and guided imagery. Now it is time to refine these skills into a very short and concise formula for reducing the pain. Today's Pain Control Imagery lesson will provide you with such a formula and your practice schedule will change slightly. You should listen to Script Number Four— The Inward Journey twice during the day. In between, practice today's autogenic formula twice an hour, every waking hour. That's a lot to ask, but if the pain control formula is going to become habitual, it must be repeated constantly. If you carry through with this repetition, then the body almost immediately will activate the formula when you experience your pain problem. This formula should be memorized; taping it is optional, but may help you in learning it.

Let's go to work.

> *Take a deep breath.*
> *Let it out slowly.*
> *Close your eyes.*
> *My arms and legs are heavy and warm.*
> *My heartbeat is calm and regular.*
> *My breathing is calm and regular.*
> *My stomach is warm.*
> *My forehead is cool.*
> *My built-in painkiller is working.*
> (Repeat five times.)
>
> *Painkillers flow to all parts of my body.*
> (Repeat five times.)
>
> *My body blocks the pain.*
> (Repeat five times.)
>
> *Time to end the exercise.*
> *Take a deep breath, let it out slowly and open your eyes.*
> *Flex your arms and legs.*
> *Wide awake and pain-free.*

NOTE: If you find that phrasing the statement slightly differently to suit your particular needs helps you achieve better pain control without changing the intent of the formula, feel free to make the alteration. The Internal Pain Block is to be used whenever you see a Pain Sticker and, as the Pain Control Imagery, is to be practiced two minutes out of every waking hour.

PAIN BONUS: LEISURE ACTIVITIES

Develop a hobby to get your mind off the pain!

If you develop a leisure activity that focuses your energies on something other than your pain, your perception of pain diminishes. Recognizing a sound idea and implementing it don't always go together.

The answer to the question of implementation lies directly with you. You are the only person who truly knows what gives you enjoyment and what leisure activities are best suited to your personality, lifestyle and environment.

Requirements

A good leisure activity should be one that:

- You would like to repeat on a regular basis.
- Provides you with a sense of enjoyment.
- Is economically feasible.
- Provides you with a sense of satisfaction.
- Does not exceed your physical limitations.
- May involve members of your family or friends.
- Has no age limitations and can be continued for as long as you like.

These Aren't Hobbies

Not all people have the same conception of what a leisure activity involves, so I have included a list of nonproductive "hobbies."

- Smoking.
- Watching television for hours a day.
- Complaining about the world economic situation.
- Complaining about politics.
- Talking about your pain.
- Talking about other people's pain.
- Staying in bed all day.
- Being angry at everyone.

For the sake of time and space, I have tried to keep the list short, but each of these has been given to me as a leisure activity by my patients!

Developing Your Leisure Activity

The first step in developing good leisure activities for yourself will be to take the Leisure Inventory and develop a list of leisure activities. On a sheet of paper use this scale to rate your interest in the following activities:

4 = Extremely interested
3 = Moderately interested
2 = Can take it or leave it
1 = No interest

Stamp collecting	Photography
Walking	Tennis
Jogging	Bowling
Knitting	Needlework
Painting	Coin collecting
Plane models	Woodworking
Gardening	Hiking
Rock collecting	Astronomy
Writing	Volunteer work
Playing cards	Automobile repair
Flying	Collecting things
Crafts	Bicycling
Music	CB or ham radio
Dancing	Golf
Pets	Jewelry making

Add your own

In your notebook list all those activities you rated three and four, and combine them into one list of no more than eight activities, with the most desirable at the top, then the second most desirable, third most desirable and so on through the eight choices.

There you have it. A list of leisure activities in the order in which you can begin to investigate them.

Coming up with the list wasn't as hard as you thought it would be, was it? Now you need to use it!

PERSONAL PAIN DIAGRAM

Copy the body outlines on page 161 into your notebook and fill in. Compare with the diagram you made before the program started.

PAIN GRAPH

The final assignment for today will be to plot your pain ratings for the first week. Copy the blank graph into your notebook and use the week's scores to mark your progress.

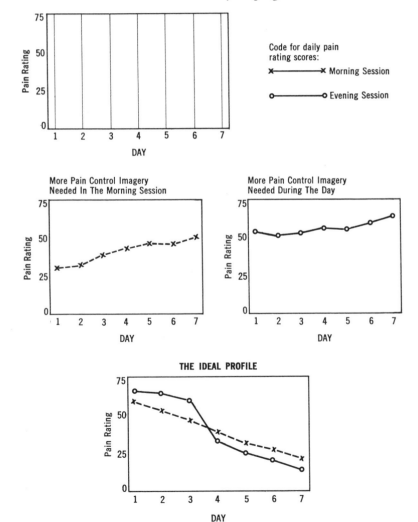

17

❧

Pain Control Program: Week Two

The final seven days of the Pain Control Program launch you into the Pain Imagery Formula. This formula is the key to your sending endorphins to any pain site in the body. Here is the setup for Day Eight through Day Fourteen.

All practice sessions are twice a day, each lasting thirty minutes. Your specialized pain formula should be practiced at least two minutes out of every waking hour. Every hour may seem like a lot of time, but add it up: twelve hours times two minutes equals twenty-four minutes. Not much of an investment to learn control of your pain. The Personal Pain Formula is also to be used with the Pain Stickers. (See page 198.)

The Setup

Each day of the second week you will be assigned specific tasks during the morning and evening sessions. Here's the setup for each day:

- Physical Reconditioning (twice daily)
- Pain Control Imagery
    —Daily Review (once daily)
    —Personal Pain Formula (twice daily)
- Record Keeping (twice daily)

Now let's take an in-depth look at each part of your daily assignment.

PHYSICAL RECONDITIONING

The exercises are to be continued twice a day. The number of repetitions for each exercise will increase until Day Ten, then remain the same. If you want to increase them further, add no more than one repetition per day.

PAIN CONTROL IMAGERY

During each of the remaining seven days you'll be asked to perform two Pain Control Imagery sessions daily. The morning session will consist of a Daily Review and Personal Pain Formula, whereas the evening session will involve only the Personal Pain Formula.

DAILY REVIEW

Once a day you'll be asked to review a specific script from Week One. This may be done any time during the day.

PERSONAL PAIN FORMULA

This is the core of the Pain Control Program and provides you with a Pain Control Imagery formula for your specific pain.
Your personal pain formula is to be practiced during:

1. Morning session.
2. Evening session.
3. Two minutes every hour.
4. With Pain Stickers.

RECORD KEEPING

Use the Daily Record for Week Two to keep track of your progress. Copy the form below into your notebook. I've tried to keep each session as short as possible, but a full commitment to pain control require some readjustments in your lifestyle.

DAY

		8	9	10	11	12	13	14
MORNING	Physical Reconditioning							
	Daily Review							
	P.P.F.*							
	Record of Medication							
	Pain Rating							
EVENING	Physical Reconditioning							
	P.P.F.*							
	Record of Medication							
	Pain Rating							
	Optional Walk/Run							

* Personal Pain Formula

Before you start Week Two, I want to share with you two problems that could interfere with your Pain Control Program. The hurry-up personality and pain depression need to be totally eliminated—beginning today.

The Hurry-Up Personality

It may take only three seconds to cause an injury, but to resolve the pain that follows may take many years. Some people are in such a hurry that they lose the effect of the Pain Control Program by virtue of the fact that they are "hurry-up persons" and never spend enough time adequately learning the skills. If you think you might be a "hurry-up person," it would pay for you to slow down. The second week of the fourteen-day Pain Control Program was not designed to be a race.

How many of the following behavior patterns commonly associated with the "hurry-up personality" apply to you?

- Eating rapidly.
- Drinking rapidly.
- Walking rapidly.
- Talking rapidly.
- Writing your signature hurriedly.
- Reading hurriedly without good comprehension.
- Being under constant pressure at home and/or at work.
- Chronic sense of time urgency.

If you've checked any of these, you need to slow down and take your time to learn the Personal Pain Formula. Slow, sure steps will be more beneficial in the long run and will leave you with a solid base of pain control.

How Can You Tell When Pain Depression Strikes?

All of us are depressed at some time during our lives, but people who suffer from chronic pain may experience long, deep depressions that are a significant roadblock to becoming "pain-free." Most physical and emotional functions are affected by depression; if depression *should* become partner to chronic pain, then the suffering will surely increase.

First you must determine whether depression is a partner to your pain experience. Read through the list of statements provided below. How many of them apply to you when you are in pain?

DEPRESSION CHECKLIST

1. Do you fatigue easily without strenuous exercise?
2. Do you have trouble going to sleep and maintaining sleep?
3. Do you have an inability to concentrate?
4. Do you feel guilty about your pain?

5. Do you find yourself becoming indecisive?
6. Do you have a decreased feeling of affection toward loved ones?
7. Do you experience a reduced sexual interest?
8. Have you noticed an increase in your level of tension or anxiety?
9. Has there been an increase in your irritability?
10. Have you had any thoughts of suicide?
11. Is the thought of dying on your mind a great portion of time?

If you have answered Yes to any two questions, you may be allowing depression to rear its ugly head in the midst of your chronic pain.

Admitting to depression is just the first step; the second is to gain relief by following your personal Pain Control Formula. You may always refer back to the exercise on overcoming depression found in Chapter Three.

Personal Pain Formula

It's time for real excitement, for you are going to develop your Personal Pain Formula. You will repeat this formula a specified number of times during each morning and evening session. Along with your sessions, the Personal Pain Formula is to be used with the Pain Stickers.

A COMBINATION

The Personal Pain Formula (P.P.F.) is a combination of: tense/relax, autogenics, hypnosis and the inward journey. All of these techniques have been presented in Week One, and now we are going to make them into a formula for reaching your specific site of pain.

THE SECRET

The P.P.F. works because of three basic principles:

1. When physically relaxed, your brain strives to put your body into a state of equilibrium, thus reducing pain.

2. You can increase your body's production of built-in pain-killers by giving yourself internal suggestions.

3. Mental visualization of the pain site sends painkillers to the specific area.

When these three principles are combined and practiced, you will be able to control pain at any location in your body and at any time.

CUSTOMIZING YOURS

It doesn't matter whether your pain is in your lower back, foot, hand or head, the P.P.F. can apply to any area. The flexibility of your P.P.F. is unique in that you may use it for back pain today and a headache next week.

The formula consists of the basic autogenics exercise plus the personal pain insert.

THE INSERT

The phrases of your P.P.F. are to be repeated in the same manner as the autogenic phrases. Some patients have asked, "Will my brain know how much painkiller to produce and will it go to the right spot?" The answer to this complicated question is quite simple. The brain will always seek to insure body equilibrium and this means just the right amount of built-in painkiller sent to the area of discomfort. Internal suggestion and mental visualization need to be practiced intensively to insure that the brain develops the habit of quick and specific production of endorphins.

You need to be very specific regarding the pain site. If your thumb is painful because of arthritis, then the insert should be THUMB, not hand. In the same sense, the insert for a painful foot should be FOOT, not toe.

PAIN INSERT

My brain produces painkillers.
Painkillers are flowing to my _____(insert pain site)_____ .
My _____(insert pain site)_____ is becoming pain-free.
I am controlling the pain in my _____(insert pain site)_____ .

The Personal Pain Formula

Each session will consist of repeating the Personal Pain Formula a specified number of times. Remember to begin by assuming a comfortable position, taking three deep breaths and letting them out slowly, closing your eyes and repeating the phrases silently to yourself. Terminate each session by flexing your arms and legs, taking a deep breath, opening your eyes and getting up slowly.

Assume your relaxed position. Repeat each of the Personal Pain Formula phrases, silently to yourself.

My arms and legs are heavy and warm.
My heartbeat is calm and regular.
My breathing is calm and regular.
My stomach is warm.
My forehead is cool.
My brain produces painkillers.
Painkillers are flowing to my _____ (insert pain site) _____ .
My _____ (insert pain site) _____ is becoming pain-free.
I am controlling the pain in my _____ (insert pain site) _____ .

Time to terminate this exercise.
Flex your arms and legs.
Take a deep breath.
Open your eyes and sit up slowly.

NOTE: When practicing the Personal Pain Formula during the day, you may eliminate the eye closing.

Remember, the effectiveness of your Personal Pain Formula is increased if you visualize the pain site as vividly as possible, thus helping your brain direct the endorphins to the pain site.

LET'S PUT THE P.P.F. TO GOOD USE. START DAY EIGHT!

TODAY'S ASSIGNMENT

- Physical Reconditioning (twice)
- Pain in Control Imagery
  —Daily Review (once)
  —Personal Pain Formula (twice)
- Record Keeping—after each morning and evening session

PHYSICAL RECONDITIONING

Do all ten exercises each morning and evening session.

1. Head Rolls: five right, five left
2. Shoulders Up and Down: ten
3. Arm Circles: twelve forward, twelve backward
4. Back Stretcher: twelve
5. Back Bender: eight right, eight left
6. Pelvic Tilt: four
7. Single Knee to Chest: eight each leg
8. Double Knee to Chest: eight
9. Curl Downs: six
10. Curl Ups: six

MORNING SESSION   *Time:* **60 Minutes**

- Physical Reconditioning
- Daily Review
    Start the P.C.I. session off right with a review of the Autogenics tape from Day Three.
- Personal Pain Formula

Here is the basic core. It's up to you to practice your Personal Pain Formula fifteen times.

214

EVENING SESSION   *Time:* **40 Minutes**

· Physical Reconditioning
· Personal Pain Formula

Practice fifteen times.

TODAY'S ASSIGNMENT

- Physical Reconditioning (twice)
- Pain Control Imagery
  - —Daily Review (once)
  - —Personal Pain Formula (twice)
- Record Keeping—after each morning and evening session

NOTE: Don't forget to go back to Week One and review the Pain Bonuses.

PHYSICAL RECONDITIONING

1. Head Rolls: five right, five left
2. Shoulders Up and Down: ten
3. Arm Circles: twelve forward, twelve backward
4. Back Stretcher: twelve
5. Back Bender: eight right, eight left
6. Pelvic Tilt: five
7. Single Knee to Chest: eight each leg
8. Double Knee to Chest: eight
9. Curl Downs: six
10. Curl Ups: six

MORNING SESSION   *Time:* **65 Minutes**

- Physical Reconditioning
- Daily Review
  Take out the Inward Journey tape and review the technique.
- Personal Pain Formula
  Practice your formula fifteen times.

EVENING SESSION   *Time:* **40 Minutes**

- Physical Reconditioning
- Personal Pain Formula
   Practice fifteen times.

NOTE: Remember to use the P.P.F. two minutes out of every waking hour and when reminded by the Pain Stickers.

TODAY'S ASSIGNMENT

- Physical Reconditioning (twice)
- Pain Control Imagery
  —Daily Review (once)
  —Personal Pain Formula (twice)
- Record Keeping—after each morning and evening session

PHYSICAL RECONDITIONING

1. Head Rolls: six right, six left
2. Shoulders Up and Down: ten
3. Arm Circles: twelve forward, twelve backward
4. Back Stretcher: fourteen
5. Back Bender: ten right, ten left
6. Pelvic Tilt: five
7. Single Knee to Chest: ten each leg
8. Double Knee to Chest: eight
9. Curl Downs: six
10. Curl Ups: six

MORNING SESSION   *Time:* 60 Minutes

- Physical Reconditioning
- Daily Review
  Listen to Script Number Three—Autogenics again.
- Personal Pain Formula
  Practice twenty times.

EVENING SESSION   *Time:* 45 Minutes

- Physical Reconditioning
- Personal Pain Formula
  Practice twenty times.

TODAY'S ASSIGNMENT

· Physical Reconditioning (twice)
· Pain Control Imagery
  —Daily Review (optional)
  —Personal Pain Formula (twice)
· Record Keeping—after each morning and evening session

PHYSICAL RECONDITIONING

At this point you have reached the peak of physical reconditioning for the two-week program. Stay at this level for the remaining four days. During the Maintenance Program, you may increase the repetitions for an exercise, but by no means more than one additional repetition per exercise per day.

MORNING SESSION   *Time:* **45 Minutes**

· Physical Reconditioning (Follow the schedule for Day Ten)
· Daily Review (Optional)
  While the Daily Review is optional from now on in the program, you will find listening to the tapes from Week One of great benefit.
· Personal Pain Formula
  Practice twenty times.

EVENING SESSION   *Time:* **45 Minutes**

· Physical Reconditioning (Day Ten schedule)
· Personal Pain Formula
  Practice twenty times.

TODAY'S ASSIGNMENT

- Physical Reconditioning (twice)
- Pain Control Imagery
   —Daily Review (once)
   —Personal Pain Formula (twice)
- Record Keeping—after each morning and evening session

MORNING SESSION   *Time:* **35 Minutes**

- Physical Reconditioning (Day Ten schedule)
- Daily Review (Optional)
- Personal Pain Formula
   Practice twenty times.

EVENING SESSION   *Time:* **35 minutes**

- Physical Reconditioning (Day Ten schedule)
- Personal Pain Formula
   Practice twenty times.

TODAY'S ASSIGNMENT

- Physical Reconditioning (twice)
- Pain Control Imagery
  —Personal Pain Formula (twice)
- Record Keeping—after each session

MORNING SESSION   *Time:* 35 Minutes

- Physical Reconditioning (Day Ten schedule)
- Daily Review (Optional)
- Personal Pain Formula
  Practice twenty times.

EVENING SESSION   *Time:* 35 Minutes

- Physical Reconditioning (Day Ten schedule)
- Personal Pain Formula
  Practice twenty times.

TODAY'S ASSIGNMENT

- Physical Reconditioning (twice)
- Pain Control Imagery
  —Personal Pain Formula (twice)
- Record Keeping—after each session
- Review
- Personal Pain Diagram (page 161)
- Pain Influence Scale (page 21)
- Pain Graph (page 206)

MORNING SESSION   *Time:* 40 Minutes

- Physical Reconditioning (Day Ten schedule)
- Daily Review (Optional)
- Personal Pain Formula
  Practice twenty-five times.

EVENING SESSION   *Time:* 40 Minutes

- Physical Reconditioning (Day Ten schedule)
- Personal Pain Formula
  Practice twenty-five times.

A Not-So-Final Word

Although you've reached the last day of the two-week Pain Control Program, your work has just begun. It's time to begin the Maintenance Program.

Most people need further practice to increase the effectiveness of their pain control skills. The more frequently you practice your Personal Pain Formula, the better you will be able to control any pain at any time.

Congratulate yourself! But don't stop—go on to the Maintenance Program. You've only begun to gain POWER OVER YOUR PAIN WITHOUT DRUGS.

PART III

18

❧

Your Maintenance Program

The Maintenance Program is just what the word implies—you will maintain your practice of the Pain Control Program, but on a somewhat reduced level. No one becomes 100 percent proficient at all of the pain control skills during the fourteen-day period, so the Maintenance Program is designed to help you keep your present skill level and increase the potency of your pain control techniques.

Follow these simple steps:

STEP ONE: Set practice sessions in the morning or evening. In the Maintenance Program you have only *one* session a day. It is essential that you continue practicing whether at home, on vacation or anywhere you may be. Skipping even one day can set back your Maintenance Program. Remember, pain is always looking for an excuse to return.

STEP TWO: Continue to record each day's activities in the Daily Record. This will serve as a positive reinforcer.

Some Common Questions

QUESTION: *How long will I have to continue the maintenance program?*

ANSWER: The Pain Control Imagery must be practiced each day along with the physical reconditioning.

225

QUESTION: *If I feel good one day, can I skip my pain control practice?*

ANSWER: Absolutely not. Pain Control Imagery is a skill that needs to be practiced every day. As you become more proficient, the amount of time you need to practice will be less and less, but never skip a day.

QUESTION: *Should I continue to see my doctor?*

ANSWER: Yes. The Pain Control Program is not a substitute for proper medical treatment.

QUESTION: *Can I substitute the exercise for walk/run?*

ANSWER: Yes, but check with your doctor first. Since running and riding the exercycle are very similar, make sure to start your program at a low level and work yourself up gradually. See exercycle chart in Appendix II.

QUESTION: *Will the pain control be permanent?*

ANSWER: It will stay with you as long as you practice and have the desire to control your discomfort.

Just the Beginning

That's right, the fourteen-day Pain Control Program was just the start. What you do from this point on will determine whether you are going to maintain POWER OVER YOUR PAIN WITHOUT DRUGS. No one ever promised you a pain-free rose garden. Hard work, determination and a positive attitude are still your best weapons in the battle against pain. The Maintenance Program was developed to give you the best opportunity for achieving success.

Learning pain control is not an easy task; it takes courage, perseverance and true commitment to become well again. I know what you've gone through is difficult because I've taken the journey myself. But no pain problem is hopeless. I have yet to work with a patient who could not learn to decrease his or her pain to some degree if he or she had the will to do so. And the fact that you stayed with me through this book indicates that you have that motivation—so I know you will win out!

APPENDIX I

◈

INFORMATION ABOUT PAIN CLINICS

Because of the great proliferation of pain centers in the United States, there should be one in your geographical area. The fact that an organization, hospital or group of people call themselves a pain clinic (or some such name) is no measure of the quality of their practice. The American Association of Anesthesiologists, 515 Busse Highway, Park Ridge, IL 60068 will send you a list of pain clinics.

Since there are no national certification criteria for pain clinics, here is a form you should use when inquiring about them.

Pain Clinic Checklist

You can evaluate a pain clinic by checking it out against the questions below. If the answer to any question is No, that clinic may not be for you.

1. Are licensed physicians on the staff?
2. Is there a physical and psychological evaluation required before entering clinic?
3. Are licensed psychologists or psychiatrists on the staff?
4. Is exercise part of the program?
5. Are previous patients available for you to talk to?
6. Can you tour the clinic?
7. Is there a follow-up or maintenance program?
8. Are exact cost figures available to you?

9. Is there a drug withdrawal process in the program?
10. Will they allow you to take your time in making a decision?

Last of all, don't make a snap decision. Think about your choice, gather all of the information and then make a very considered decision.

NOTE: Be wary of any clinic that is quick to give out guarantees of instantaneous results and miracle cures.

APPENDIX II

OPTIONAL EXERCYCLE PROGRAM

The optional exercycle program is designed to be totally compatible with your Pain Control Program. Keep track of time and total distance in your notebook. Once you have reached Day Eleven, continue this time and distance for Days Twelve, Thirteen and Fourteen, and throughout the Maintenance Program. Each assignment is to be practiced *four* times daily.

DAILY ASSIGNMENTS

Day One	=	5 min. at 8 MPH
Day Two	=	6 min. at 8 MPH
Day Three	=	7 min. at 9 MPH
Day Four	=	8 min. at 10 MPH
Day Five	=	9 min. at 11 MPH
Day Six	=	10 min. at 11 MPH
Day Seven	=	10 min. at 12 MPH
Day Eight	=	11 min. at 12 MPH
Day Nine	=	12 min. at 13 MPH
Day Ten	=	12 min. at 14 MPH
Day Eleven	=	12 min. at 15 MPH
Day Twelve	=	12 min. at 15 MPH

If at any time you want to increase the duration and/or speed of your riding, do so in a very gradual manner. A good rule of thumb is not to increase your riding more than one minute or one mile per hour per day.

Index